VANILLA TO KINKY

THE BEGINNER'S GUIDE TO BDSM AND KINK

Transform your boring sex life with BDSM and Learn the Keys to How to be Dominant or Submissive in the Bedroom

by

Jonathan Wolf

Contents

Free Questionnaire

Are you a Dom? a sub? or maybe a switch?

Not exactly sure where you are on the BDSM spectrum?

No problem, let's figure it out.

visit:

Vanillatokinky.com

For your **free, instant result, 3-minute questionnaire.**

Hope it helps!

INTRODUCTION

♥ ♥ ♥

How many times have we heard someone say, "This is going to change your life?" It seems to have become a weekly occurrence. Whether it's the new Hollywood blockbuster, the new hit show with a cult following, or gluten-free cupcakes, a lot of things promise to change our lives. I believe the only things that can truly change our lives have to do with our health. I'm not talking about a fad diet or a 200-page book that boils down to being more positive, I'm talking about quality, fundamental changes to the way we live. To genuinely improve the quality of our lives, we have to be willing and able to make changes. We have to reframe our attitudes towards the world and those around us. We have to analyze who we interact with and how we interact with them. A good hard look at our diet cannot hurt things either. And most important of all, we must have higher quality sex. High five!

Like lava lamps, sex is strange yet fascinating. In the 90's it started very young, usually in a classroom where the teacher put a video on and stepped out to smoke a cigarette.

Nowadays, we learn everything about sex from wiki-articles, Pornhub, and clumsy experiences in high school and college. We live in this society where many of us are completely hypnotized by sex while it is simultaneously considered taboo to even discuss it. It's 20 freaking 19, I think it's about time we become a little more open about sex.

Like fast food french fries, sex is sometimes hot and delicious, while other times it is cold, stale, and you regret it afterwards. There is no reason you should be having crappy. It is 20-freakin'-19, you have the right and the dignity to expect quality sex from your partner. You shouldn't have to lay there miserable while someone works you over like you owe money to a casino. Or maybe you do owe money, and crappy sex isn't be your most immediate problem. My point is, crappy sex should NEVER be the norm. In *Vanilla to Kinky—The Beginner's Guide to BDSM and Kink*, we are going to have a very frank and open discussion about sex. This is a shame-free zone. As long as you follow the golden rule of safe-sane-consensual, then there is nothing to be ashamed of in your sexual desires.

One of the challenges in discussing BDSM is getting past this universal taboo of discussing. How can we discuss kinky sex if we get hung up just broaching the subject? I am not going to pull any punches with you. By the end of this book, you will be more comfortable around sex. You will feel confident in your newfound knowledge, you will be able to raise the topic of sex with your friends, and you will be able to convey your needs to your partner or partners.

I have this philosophy about sex where our sexual identity is the truest part of who we are. I'm not talking liking guys, girls, or both, I'm talking about the specific things you desire during sex. When you're in a sexual situation, all pretenses must leave the room immediately. If you have to be a tough SOB because you're in a leadership position at work, if you have to be constantly focused because your job is stressful, if you have to be constantly attentive because your job requires intimate care, you can simply cast those responsibilities away in the bedroom. If you have to be a dutiful son or daughter for your parents, if you have to be a stern mother or father for your rowdy children, if you have to be responsible and wise for your siblings, you can throw that out in the bedroom. So much of our lives is putting on this mask and pretending to be something we aren't just function, and it is stressful, and it causes us to lose sight of who we are. Through the teachings and practices of BDSM you will gain the knowledge of who you really are, as well as be given the permission to act on your true identity.

Supposed you're the perfect wife and daughter. You work hard, take care of everything, keep the house, call your mom every Sunday. You're the perfect woman everyone wants you to be. But maybe, you want to be spanked. Maybe you want to be punished because you don't think you're good enough, maybe you want to be guilty of something and have your partner discipline you. That is completely normal and healthy. BDSM gives you a safe and effective way to explore those feelings without causing emotional or physical damage. You're allowed to be that naughty girl.

Maybe you're just a great guy. You volunteer, donate to charity, coach little league. You take care of your partner and make sure they know they're loved and cared for. You're almost too perfect. But you have a dark side. You love hardcore porn. You view it for hours. You frequently masturbate to hurting women during sex. Of course, you don't want to rape anyone or injure someone in real life, but the fantasy is so engrossing you can't stop looking at the porn. That's normal. You're allowed to have sadistic fantasies. You can even carry them out with a willing partner. Sex and shame should never, ever mix. You're allowed to want those dark things.

There are endless amounts of kinks and sexual desires. Sexual desires are as unique as the person having them. Some people want to be tied up during sex. Some want to be helpless; some just want their hands tied, some people want to be tied up where others can see them. Except for asexuals, everyone has their own unique kinks. And the most screwed up thing ever is 99% of sexual desires are considered weird or abnormal. That's stupid. That is the most asinine thing ever concocted. Let me be perfectly frank, all sexual desires are completely acceptable no matter what. You are allowed to have any sexual desire you want, even if it is taboo or illegal. Whether you act on it or not is a completely different story. Remember the golden rule. If your fantasy is safe, sane, and consensual, then it is okay to act on it.

While BDSM has a very specific meaning, it really is just a set of teachings and practices to help you explore your sexuality safely and intelligently. No acronym can completely encompass every kink under the sun, but the activities listed in **B**ondage and Discipline, **D**omination and Submission, **S**adism and **M**asochism encompass the vast majority of kinks and fantasies. No one is asking you to buy a leather corset or get your butt whipped (though if you like that, all the power to you). This is a journey of sexual exploration. You are going to receive a broad understanding of the wide world of sexuality. You will learn about the sexual paradigms present in BDSM, and which ones suit your tastes. The most important thing you can do is enter with an open mind and explore your sexual education after you finish the book.

Imagine if you read one cooking article in a magazine and based the rest of your meals around that. That would be ridiculous. Our sexuality is an ever-evolving thing. Many people find that as they become more comfortable with the entry level stuff, they start to crave more "taboo" and interesting things. That's fine. As long as your life remains safe, sane, and consensual, you can crave whatever you want. Exploring BDSM for the first time is like discovering a new and exciting regional cuisine that you have never experienced in your life. By reading this book, you have started on a thrilling new chapter of your life.

I find sexual satisfaction to be supremely important to a content life. Even if you're just having sex by yourself, you can still have a satisfying sex life. As long as you get to engage in your true kinks and desires, even by proxy, you will be more content in your life. Have you ever had a sweet craving? Could you imagine if you eating potato chips every night for months on end, even years on end, when all you want is a sweet treat? It's the same as if you have a deep-seated sexual desire you're not allowed to explore. You shouldn't subject yourself to that (unless you're into sexual denial which can be very hot).

In *Vanilla to Kinky—The Beginner's Guide to BDSM and Kink*, we are going to explore the fundamentals of **B**ondage and **D**iscipline, **D**omination and **S**ubmission, **S**adism and **M**asochism and how they apply to you. That certainly doesn't mean you have to find every single thing kinky. Many people just gravitate towards a single aspect of BDSM, and that's totally acceptable. Remember what I said earlier about your bedroom experiences; this isn't about having another set of expectations laid at your feet. This is about discovering who you are as a sexual being. This is about happiness and satisfaction. So many health and wellness books are about making difficult changes in your life. They're about new responsibilities and restrictions. This experience is going to be the complete opposite. You are going to learn new freedoms and new ways to enjoy yourself. All you must do is keep an open mind and a thirst for exploration. So many things claim they're going to change your life. BDSM is going to change your life. You will be freer and happier than you have ever been. You will learn things about yourself that you never knew before. Socrates, arguably the greatest philosopher who ever lives, said the unexamined life is not worth living. You are going to take an honest examination of your life and discover the things that bring you joy and satisfaction.

I can't imagine what it's like to be you right. If you're new to BDSM and sexual exploration, you have so many amazing and positive changes in store for you. You have picked up the right book. You are a sexual novice taking the first step to sexual enlightenment. You're unlocking more depth and complexity to your soul than you can possibly imagine. I'm so happy I get to guide you on your journey. Pardon my French, but this is a fucking awesome journey you're about to go on. I feel like I'm standing outside your rocket ship and you're about to be launched to the moon. I have found that sexual exploration is one of the most rewarding things in life. It's like discovering a new favorite TV show or a new favorite food. It's about indulging your soul.

It's not just about orgasms. BDSM is about identifying and satisfying these primal, animal needs in your brain stem. It's intense. You might become cum drunk, which we'll discuss later on. You're not going to just have awesome orgasms and experiences, but you'll notice that satisfying these primordial sexual urges just makes your life better. You're less stressed, more focused, more outgoing. You're just more comfortable in your own skin after you learn these new exciting things about yourself.

Vanilla to Kinky—The Beginner's Guide to BDSM and Kink breaks down as follows. First you will learn exactly what BDSM is and how it applies to every single person's sexuality, including your own. We'll go through common terms and histories as well as help you find exactly where you are on the BDSM spectrum. Myths perpetuated in popular media will be shattered and you will learn that BDSM isn't about whips and chains but instead is about personal sexual satisfaction.

Once you have an academic understanding of BDSM theory, you will learn safe and effective sexual practices. This isn't about how to put a condom on, boys and girls. You're going to learn the safe sex techniques they didn't teach you in Sex Ed. You're going to learn how to separate BDSM from abuse. It's very easy for the uneducated to slip from Domination and submission into abuse. I'm not going to let that happen to you. You're going to learn the basics of roleplaying and how-to setup scenes to enhance your sexual fantasies. Bondage is an exciting aspect of BDSM but deadly if not done properly. You are going to learn everything you ever wanted to know about safe and effective bondage.

Toys, toys, toys! We like toys in buttttttssss! Toys, toys, toys! But seriously, you're going to get a crash course in sex toys and why they're so awesome. This includes safe and effective techniques for impact play. Finally, we will close the chapter by discussing the importance of aftercare. BDSM doesn't end with orgasms. The kind of sex you are going to have as a BDSM practitioner is going to be so intense and mind-blowing, that you're going to need to come down mentally and emotionally afterwards. This is where aftercare comes in and why it is so important. I will bring up aftercare a lot in this book because it is so damn important for a quality sexual experience.

Once you understand the theories and practices of BDSM, you are ready to launch right into the thick of things. Whether you want to bring up BDSM with your partner or find like-minded singles in your area, we got you covered. Communication is critical to a positive experience. We're going to learn how to bring it up with your partner and have a good time, once things begin. Once you understand good communication, we're going to help you find other people in

BDSM. Trust me when I say there are a lot of who live near you into the same things you are.

Finally, we will end the book with some closing words on BDSM and how it isn't right for everyone. We'll summarize what we learned and even provide a helpful cheat sheet you can refer to once the book is over.

You are ready for this. You deserve this. You deserve to be happy. You deserve quality sexual experiences that engage your kinks and fantasies. This isn't some mysterious world with dominatrix's and sex dungeons. This is an attainable reality where you have the best sex of your life. All you need is an open mind and relentless curiosity. Please take this journey with me, and know that you won't regret a thing.

PART I

ENTER THE WONDERFUL WORLD OF BDSM

♥ ♥ ♥

*C*ome with me, and you will be, in a world of sexual *emancipation.* BDSM stands for **B**ondage and **D**iscipline, **D**omination and submission, **S**adism and **M**asochism. Aside from breaking down the acronym, it's really difficult to give an exact definition of BDSM. For our purposes, BDSM is a collection of theories and practices used to explore sexuality. It is true that there are forms of BDSM that have nothing to do with eroticism, especially as it pertains to Domination and submission, but we're not going to focus on that in this book.

BDSM really incorporates the vast majority of sexuality. Almost any fantasy or kink you can think of is about bondage, discipline, domination, submission, sadism, and/or masochism. I wouldn't even call it a lifestyle choice. There's no whips or chains or people screaming at you, it's just a system used to organize and explore your sexuality. Popular media has given a very distorted view of BDSM through the years. Whenever it is depicted, it's always as a gag with

10

someone tied to the wall and someone else whipping them. There's always leather involved somehow. It's seen as a silly niche' that weirdos get into. *Fifty Shades of Grey* brought BDSM into the mainstream. I would bet there's a 50% chance you read that book before reading this book. And that's great. 50 Shades popularized the idea of exploring your sexuality, even if it fell into some of the old tropes and gives a dangerous and misguided example of a D/s relationship. For some reason, writers think there has to be a dungeon (or red room) involved when it comes to any sex besides missionary position with the lights off.

There are so many confusing notions about BDSM out there that it's excellent you took the time to actually educate yourself. They key to a quality education is understanding the fundamentals and then building off of them. If you're ever unsure about something when it comes to sex, always return to the fundamentals for guidance

The Golden Rule

Before I teach you anything, young padawan, you must first learn and understand the meaning of **safe, sane, and consensual**. This isn't something exclusive to BDSM but should be applied to all sexual activity. All sexual activity should be safe. While it is impossible to eliminate all the danger from a sexual encounter (you can still get an STD no matter how boring the sex is), you should take every reasonable step to make the experience as safe as possible as well as avoid activity that contains a reasonable chance of harm. Experienced participants in BDSM practice extreme bondage, choking, and rape-play, all of which can lead to deaths or felonies, but hopefully they practice them in such a way as to minimize the risk involved. I don't want you to feel scared entering into your first BDSM experience. When it comes to sexual encounters, there is always risk, but you can take reasonable steps to minimize risk.

There is an argument about what sane means exactly, but I think both interpretations have merit. Some believe sane means only participating in sane behavior. This ties back into safe, but also refers to avoiding situations that can lead to one or both of you being arrested (public sex, hello), avoid a situation where you become codependent and obsessed with each other to the point it causes dysfunction outside the bedroom (this can happen to emotionally dependent submissives), and avoiding threats to your physical, mental, emotional, and social wellbeing. BDSM is not a drug or an addiction. If you find yourself forsaking your personal responsibilities for sex, you need to seek professional help immediately. I know sex is amazing, especially when you discover the things that genuinely turn you on, but there's more to life than sex, like slurpees and stuff.

Sane can also mean entering into any sexual situation without emotional or mental impairment. You shouldn't drink or get high to the point you won't remember a sexual encounter the next day. I know a few drinks or a spliff (that's a marijuana) can really loosen things up in the bedroom, but when practicing things like bondage or Domination and submission, you really want to be in your full faculties. You also don't want to be in a state of mind where you're sad or angry and are using sex to remedy some wrong in your life. Having sex with a rageful person can be dangerous, and you don't to go to the bedroom so depressed that you don't care what happens to you. You should always enter a sexual situation in your full faculties.

Finally, we come to consensual. All parties should agree to everything that is happening, and everything that is planned. Surprises are awesome, especially during sex, but that can also be painful or terrifying. Clear verbal consent is critical to a positive sexual experience. This isn't about two robots giving consent every 30 seconds. Talk beforehand about the things you would like to try in the bedroom. If you want to try something new on the spur of the moment, make sure your partner is comfortable with what you're doing. The easiest way to manage this is with a safe-word (or action if you're gagged). A safe-word can be any word you want, and every participant should have one, even Dom's, tops, and sadists. It should be a unique word that wouldn't occur during sex like "cereal," "oregano," "chamomile," "potato chip," "coleslaw," (checks grocery list), or "spaghetti." It should not be an ambivalent word like "No", or "Stop." Some people like to shout "No" or "Stop" during sex because they are roleplaying in their mind. There has to be no mistake what the safe-word is and everyone involved should have it memorized.

Bondage

Bondage is the consensual practice of binding or restraining a person for the purposes of pleasure. Bondage is not simply tying someone to the bed and fucking them. You can restrain someone to inhibit or completely eliminate their movement. You can bind parts of their body like their cock or breasts. This has no effect on their movement but is solely for the pleasure of at least one participant. Blindfolding someone is also considered bondage. You are not restricting their movement, but instead, one of their senses. This can greatly heighten anticipation during sex. There are several forms of bondage and entire books have dedicated to just this aspect of BDSM.

Like all aspects of BDSM, you don't have to participate in any facet you don't enjoy. If being tied up makes you anxious or panicky, you don't have to do it. Remember, you don't have to do bondage just because it's in the acronym. You're just supposed to take the parts you enjoy and throw away the rest. This isn't like a diet where you have to strictly follow the guidelines. I told you this was going to be easy. You're going to take the parts you like and enjoy them. I highly recommend you try everything at least once, but if makes you uncomfortable, you don't have to do it. Don't let anyone pressure you into a sexual situation that makes you uncomfortable.

To help inspire you, I'm going to list several forms of bondage and their purpose. It would be impossible for me to list them all, so I'm going to stick with the most common one. The most common is probably restraining someone's hands. In the next chapter we will go into the specifics of doing this safely as there is a serious risk of blood clots when done improperly. Also bear in mind that bondage isn't just about being bound but also binding your partner. Just because you identify as male or female doesn't mean you have to find any specific thing arousing. Every person is different. Now as far as binding hands goes, this can create an intense sense of defenseless. You can feel like you're at the whims of your partner, unable to defend yourself from their sexual advances. This can be combined with binded feet to make you or your partner truly helpless. At the most extreme, people can be suspended from the ceiling by the material binding them. In this fashion they can be put on display for their partner or an audience, and conceivably be used as a sex toy.

Blindfolding is another common form of bondage. Sight is our most reliable and used sense, and without it we are helpless. The most intense part of being blindfolded can be the anticipation of what will happen next and when will it happen. This can be combined with earplugs or headphones, severely limiting the victim's ability to sense their partner in the area.

While it may not seem like it, binding is another form of bondage. The most common ways to bind a person are a woman's breasts or a man's cock. When a woman has her breasts bound, she can have feeling of helplessness, or feel like or breasts are being put on display for others. The pressure of the material against the breasts can also be highly pleasurable. Special cages have been invented to bind a man's cock. This prevents him from receiving any penal stimulation or achieving an erection. A man can become completely dependent on his partner to be released from his chastity.

In addition to tradition restraints and bindings, you can also keep your partner in a cage. This is an excellent way to achieve things like Domination or pet play. Some people enjoy feeling like a reliant sex pet towards their partner while others may enjoy the animalistic feelings of being kept in a cage, only to be let out during sex.

Discipline

Discipline is interesting because it truly ties into all other aspects of BDSM. Domination and submission are intimately tied to discipline, and bondage and sadism are ways of enforcing it. At its core, discipline is the modification or control of another person's behavior through punishment or threat of punishment. Sometimes the point of discipline is to break the rules set before you in order to immerse yourself in feelings of guilt or shame. Other times, the point of discipline is to allow another person to take control of you, or to take control of your partner. Conversely, discipline can be created through positive reinforcement, rewarding your partner with sexual favors.

The punishments and favors involved in BDSM are truly limitless and it would be impossible to list them all. I will detail several popular ones to give you inspiration for your own sexual adventures. One of the most primal forms of discipline is spanking. Spanking is a great tool for experimenting with BDSM. By putting someone over your knee (or vice versa) you are participating in light bondage. Spanking is a part of sadomasochism, and taking a spanking is a form of submission. Bear in mind when I discuss these activities, all of them can go both ways. You can inflict or receive the spankings in your relationship, or switch back and forth depending on what mood you are in. There is a very low risk of injury during spankings, though prolonged spankings can lead to broken skin. The flat of your butt generally has a reasonable pain tolerance, and it is very easy to control how soft or hard you spank someone. As a bonus, spanking seems to be a trope in our cultural awareness. Spanking is so synonymous with correction and bad behavior, that you might have a sub-conscious response to giving or receiving a spanking.

Aside from spankings, there are tons of things you can do to enforce discipline. There are tons of toys and tools that are great for punishment. Whips, rods, crops, canes, and floggers are all common toys used for discipline. As you can see, all the parts of BDSM overlap at times. Everything we are talking about here is intimately tied to sadism and masochism. Any of these devices can be focused on most of parts of the body, the breasts, butt, and genitals being the most common.

Discipline isn't just about correction through. It's using punishment to correct any behavior. Other forms of discipline include denial or verbal abuse. You can correct behavior by not allowing the submissive to orgasm or even touch themselves. If they find it erotic, you can also insult them and call them degrading names. Don't feel guilty because you like being called a slut or a whore during sex. You're allowed to enjoy stuff like that. Remember, BDSM is about stripping away these pretenses and responsibilities forced on us. We're trying to get to a place where we push that facade aside and indulge our truest desires. If you want to act like a huge whore in the bedroom, you go for it. As long as you remain safe, sane, and consensual, this is your pleasure to achieve.

Discipline is often used to teach a submissive person how to be properly submissive, but it can also be used as simple foreplay. Sometimes the most erotic part is breaking the rules set for you. Just be sure you and your partner are on the same page. Some Dominants take discipline very seriously, and you absolutely do not want any miscommunications about what is expected of you.

Domination

This is the aspect of BDSM I definitely have the most experience with. Domination is about being the active and controlling person in the sexual encounter. Anyone can be the Dominant person at any time, though it is a massive struggle for both people to be Dominant simultaneously. Your gender has no bearing on whether you are Dominant or not. Men can submissive, and women can be Dominant. You can swap roles during the encounter or on different nights as long as both of you are enjoying the experience.

Domination isn't about total control though. Things can get very confusing when explaining the Dominant/submissive dynamic. The Dominant controls the submissive but must respect any rules and limits the submissive sets. A limit is any behavior or action prohibited during sex. Almost everyone has limits, and limits should be honored at all times. There are things called soft limits and hard limits though. Soft limits are things generally prohibited during a sexual encounter but can be attempted if your partner is sufficiently aroused. Hard limits are actions forbidden under any and all circumstances. It is wise to discuss limits with your partner before any sexual encounter. Make no mistake, a Dominant must always respect their sub's limits despite controlling them. It is extremely inappropriate to violate a person's limits.

You may have noticed or intuited that a sub is secretly the one with the most power. This is technically true. I think the prolific dominatrix Illy Hymen explained it best when she said Domination/submission (D/s) is like Dungeons and Dragons. The submissive is like the dungeon master and the Dominant is the player. The submissive sets forth some loose guidelines, and the Dominant plays in their world. The Dominant is active, they have the agency. The submissive is passive, things are done to them.

Domination is closely attached to personality. It's simply in our nature to be Dominant or submissive, and it can completely depend on who we are interacting with. Someone who is the head of a company with tons of responsibility and control over people might actually be submissive in the bedroom. Remember, this is about discovering who you are. Just because you are a certain way outside the bedroom doesn't mean you have to fill that role in the bedroom.

And a word of advice for those who believe they're Dominant. You are helping someone fulfill their most intense sexual desires. They are giving up a massive amount of control to you, and you will respect it. They are still a human being, even if they don't want to be treated like a human being during sex. You will honor their limits, you will stop if they use their safe-word, and you will provide them with aftercare which we will go into great detail about later. This isn't about hating men or women, this isn't about taking your past frustrations out on someone, this isn't about revenge, it's about exerting control over your sexual partner. You will relish in the power you wield over your partner. But you will not abuse that power. Subs feel an intense animal attraction to Dom's. This has nothing to do with physical attractiveness and everything to do with how you carry yourself. If you demand partners to submit, if you come at strangers like you already have a pre-existing sexual relationship with them, you will get nowhere. You will carry yourself with confidence and dignity. Your natural Dominance will act like an aphrodisiac.

Submissive

Now, I know what you're thinking, *"Submissive? Isn't that a sandwich at Quiznos?"* Well first off, I don't think Quiznos is a thing anymore, so jot that down. Secondly, a submissive is the passive participant during a sexual encounter. This doesn't necessarily mean the participant who is getting penetrated. A woman can be Dominant while simultaneously getting her cervix tickled by her partner. If you didn't read the previous section, I strongly urge you to. The dynamic between Dominant and submissive can blur the lines when you take into account limits. The Dominant certainly controls the submissive, but the submissive is allowed a set of limits that their Dominant is not allowed to violate under any circumstances. In that way, a submissive secretly holds the control in the dynamic. Nothing allowed that the submissive is not okay with. But don't treat this as some cheat to get what you want in bed. Sex isn't a competition, and if it was, I already won (ha-ha). The point of BDSM is to find the sexual activities that bring you the most pleasure.

Some people feel like they need to be in complete control during sex. Others want to lay back and take it. They want to be removed from decision making because making decisions is just another thing that stresses them out. Think about it like this. When you're driving in a car, would you strongly prefer to be the one driving, or assuming your partner is competent, allow them to drive? Dominants want to drive. They always want to feel like they are in control. Submissives don't need to feel like they are in control and often feel anxiety when they have to take control or make decisions. Neither is right or wrong. Neither role is superior. The entire point is to find the role that suit you the most and embrace it. Just because you're a man doesn't mean you need to take control in the bedroom. You may be shocked to find how eager and willing your partner is to take control. On the same token, just because you are woman, that doesn't mean you automatically have to be the submissive one in the bedroom.

Don't tailor your roles to some responsibility you think you owe your partner. First, you should find out how they feel. You might end up perfectly compatible, yet you wouldn't have if you automatically assumed heteronormative roles. Second, this isn't some new responsibility you have to take on. You don't owe them a submissive or Dominant partner. No one can owe someone sex. That's why sex workers don't have layaway.

Bottomline, a submissive has things done to him or her controlled by the whims of their sexual partner. They relish in feelings of weakness and helplessness. It takes a lot of strength to be a submissive. To be able to let go and cede power to another person you trust. But any submissive will tell you, letting go is a beautiful and freeing experience.

Switch

No Mario pipes here, folks. You have to admit that it's weird in 2019 how Switch means something completely different. As far as BDSM goes, a switch is someone who can take on a Dominant or a submissive role during sex. There's not a lot to say here. A switch doesn't have to be a perfect 50/50 Dominant/submissive. They can enjoy submitting 90% of the time and Dominating 10% of the time. Some switches only submit or Dominate with certain partners or with certain genders. A lifelong Dominant can become a switch or a submissive. As long as you follow the rules of safe, sane, consensual, limits, and safe-words, there is no real wrong way to do it. You can even switch in the middle of an encounter if you want. Just because there's this huge well-defined culture of what it means to be a Dominant or submissive doesn't mean you can't swap back and forth between the two. Some people find it freeing not to commit to one paradigm. Sometimes a special person brings out the Dominant or submissive in you. Experiment. Just because you think you're a Dominant doesn't mean you can't enjoy submitting. Remember, this is about pleasure and fulfillment, not fulfilling a role or responsibility.

Sadism

Sadism is easily the most misunderstood component of BDSM alongside Domination. While Domination is largely misunderstood by those who practice it, sadism is largely misunderstood by everyone on the outside. Make no mistake, sadism is receiving pleasure from causing others mental, physical, or emotional pain. But the key point to sadism as it applies to BDSM is the infliction of pain must be consensual. If the pain isn't consensual, what you are doing is considered abuse, and often a crime. While it seems like no one could enjoy being consensually beaten, whipped, or abused during sex, I can promise you there are a lot of people who enjoy it immensely. Take something as simple as spanking for example. If you enjoy spanking your partner, that's sadism. You are inflicting pain and deriving pleasure from it. And that's completely fine. Again, there is nothing wrong with inflicting pain and punishment on your partner as long it is *consensual.*

As I stated before, no sexual fantasy is wrong or evil. The evilness only manifests when we act on fantasies that aren't safe, sane, and consensual. You're allowed to fantasize about hurting men or women. You're allowed to fantasize about raping people. It's all perfectly normal and healthy. Being raped or forced into sex is an extremely common fantasy among women to the point that 66% of all women have had that fantasy[1]. If there are women who have those fantasies, then some of them need partners who are willing and excited to act them out. One of the very worst behaviors in our culture is this shame and guilt surrounding anything sexual. Shame and guilt towards sex has no place in this century. Miley Cyrus swings naked from a wrecking ball and gets 100 million views on YouTube, but it's considered awkward to discuss kinks and fetishes with the person you're sleeping with? Get the fuck out of here with that old-world mentality.

People have sex. People masturbate. People fantasize about stuff that might seem weird, taboo, or appalling to us. We need to stop pretending it's this untouchable seedy world that doesn't exist when so many of us lead these sexually rich, internal lives we are never allowed to share. If you fantasize about hurting, disciplining, or raping people, that is fine. What you need is a sexual partner who complements your sexual needs and desires in a safe, sane, and consensual environment.

To prime the pump as it were, I'm going to give you some ideas for sadistic things you can do in the bedroom with your partner or partners. Spanking is always a great place to start. Many people have strong emotional notions towards spanking that can be triggered in a sexual situation. Spanking carries very low risk in terms of permanent damage or infection, though prolonged spanking can break the skin. Spanking can be done with the flat of your hand with a whip, cane, crop, rod, or flogger.

Breast and nipple torture are also common and enjoyable activities for sadists. Something as simple as pinching your sub's nipples can elicit an intense and immediate response. You can start with pinching then move onto pulling and twisting. You can also bite their breasts or nipples. Make sure to gradually apply pressure as to not break the skin. There are numerous toys to be used for nipple torture, the most common being clamps. Alligator clamps are ideal for people new to nipple torture. They're just like the clamps used to jumpstart cars though the mouth is covered with rubber or silicone. Behind the mouth is a screw that can prevent the clamp from closing all the way. Using the screw, you can completely control how much pressure the clamps produce. I'll cover more toys in the next section, but adjustable alligator clamps are excellent for beginners. Bear in mind all the techniques and tools used for spankings can be used for breast torture.

Sadism isn't limited to just physical pain though. Name calling is an extremely popular component during sex. It's not the minefield that sitcoms make it out to be. Remember to always discuss your intentions with your partner during sex. The bedroom is no place for sadistic surprises. Always honor their limits. This doesn't mean some clinical discussion with your partner where you both pass a contract back and forth discussing every name that is allowed. Just casually mentioned you want to try some dirty talk and name-calling and see if they're interested. For some people, sex is this opportunity to act out their fantasies of being huge sluts or porn stars. There should be no pretension during sex. If your partner wants to act like a slutty porn star during sex, help them feel like it. Don't be afraid to call your partner a slut, a bitch, your pet, or a bad girl. If it works out, you can step up your game. Try calling them a whore, a porn star, or daddy's girl. Sex is your permission to physically embrace your fantasies in real life. Always honor your partner's limits, and don't be afraid to experiment. Throw around vicious terms like cum dumpster, cum rag, human toilet, or your little sex toy. From my own experiences, I can tell you that less is more. Name calling is not a rap battle where you're trying to think of every synonym under the sun. All you're doing is helping them embrace the sexual persona they hold in their mind.

Masochism

I find masochism to be the most fascinating aspect of BDSM. While many aspects of BDSM tend to be fairly straightforward, Masochism feels like an oxymoron. How does one derive pleasure from pain? Very easily as it turns out. Make no mistake, masochism is the derivation of pleasure by having pain inflicted upon you. This pain can be mental, emotional, or physical. The most common question has to be, why do masochists experience pleasure from pain. There are two schools of thought regarding the mechanisms behind masochism, neither of which need to be mutually exclusive from one another. When you experience any kind of pain, your body releases a group of hormones called endorphins which act as a natural pain killer. Some people are very sensitive to endorphins and can feel a minor buzz or even an intense sense of euphoria when pain is administered in the correct amounts. You are quite literally getting high on your own supply of hormones.

The other mechanism revolves around satisfying unconscious thoughts of guilt or shame in the form of punishment. Even people who lead good, decent lives can have a secret sense of shame or guilt they carry around, even if those feelings are not attached to any specific thing. When they experience pain or humiliation, it satisfies that sense of guilt or shame as a catharsis. There's no wrong way to enjoy masochism. As long as sexual activity remains safe, sane, and consensual, you're fine.

In my own experiences, dealing with masochists can be an intensely emotional experience. Communication is key as too much punishment can become overwhelming. Tears are often involved though tears often mean you're doing your job correctly. Please communicate with your partner as much as possible. Discuss both your intentions beforehand. Check in during sex to make sure you are both okay. And for the love of god, do aftercare. Especially after an intense session of pain and humiliation, whoever the masochist is needs affection and attention. We'll detail all the finer points of aftercare in the next chapter, but it is something you are simply not allowed to skip.

To give you some general ideas of fun things masochists can do, I strongly urge you to refer to the Sadism section of this chapter. As far as things masochists can do alone, nipple torture is common and easy, and only requires one hand. There are numerous varieties of nipple clamps you can buy, and I recommend that beginners start with adjustable alligator clamps to control how much pressure they feel. If you don't have access to nipple clamps or feel too embarrassed to order them (you already bought a book on BDSM, it's time to live a little) you can use clothespins, pliers, stay-fresh chip clips, or an adjustable wrench. When using tools, please purchase new tools just for in the bedroom. You don't want a dirty, rusty tool coming into contact with broken skin.

Body writing is also another popular thing masochist's can do alone or with a partner. simply take a marker and draw something mean on yourself, preferably on your chest. I never recommend body writing on the face as sometimes it can stain the skin. Remember when taking pictures or using a webcam that body writing in the mirror will make secrets and insults come out backwards. To remove marker, simply dab cotton balls or paper towel with nail polish remover and wipe gently then finish with soap and water. Acetone can even remove permanent marker from skin. If you're feeling bold, you can write insults or secrets on places people can't see and walk around all day knowing it's still written on your body.

Lesser Understood Roles

While I think we have a strong understanding of what a Dominant, submissive, sadist, and masochist are, there is still some misconception about what a top and a bottom are, and where any of us fit in this hierarchy. There are also more esoteric roles like master, slave, caregiver, little, voyeur, cuckold, exhibitionist, and Gooner. We have a lot to get through so if you have to go to the bathroom, do it now.

To put it simply, **tops** penetrate their partners during sex. Some people argue that a top is the dominant person during sex, but there is a thing called a **service top** where that person is essentially submissive to their bottom. Top is generally only used when describing a same sex relationship, though partners are free to switch between the top and bottom role.

A **bottom** is the one who is penetrated during sex. This can be the man or the woman, and doesn't necessarily refer to the passive partner. Power bottoms exist, and they can be very aggressive, dictating how frantic they are penetrated with the movement. Again, bottom is a role usually reserved for homosexual couples as saying things like, "Who's the guy and girl in the relationship?" ignores the complexity of personality.

A **master** is a Dominant who has complete and total control over their submissive. This role does not fit neatly into the BDSM paradigm as a Dominant must always acknowledge the limits and safe-word of their submissive. To say a submissive could have no limits is a bit misguided as there are fantasies that involve snuff (death) mutilation, and non-sexual bodily excretions.

A **slave** is really the idea of a submissive with no limits. As stated previously, the idea of having no sexual limits is a bit naive. More appropriately, a slave is a sub who has surrendered a vast portion of control to their Dominant. This surrender can last for months or years at a time.

Caregiver carries a special notation in the BDSM community. Some couples enjoy an elaborate and sustained roleplay scenario where one partner is an adult and the other partner behaves as a child for most intents and purposes. It's important not to instantly dismiss kinks and fetishes because you find them personally distasteful. DD/lg (Dom Daddy and little girl) always, ALWAYS involves two or more consenting adults. No one is being hurt. No one is harming children. It is simply an elaborate roleplay scenario.

A **little** is the adult person(s) who acts as the underage character in a DD/lg roleplay. Again, I emphasize that a little is always a consenting adult. As I've stated previously, no kink or fetish is harmful if it is not acted upon. We have no control over what things make our body respond sexually. All we can do is choose whether or not we act on them. If two consenting adults are behaving safe, sane, and consensual, who are we to even give our negative input?

To put it simply, a **voyeur** is someone who likes to watch. This can really be watching anything. You might enjoy watching people undress or take a shower. You might enjoy watching people have sex or masturbate. You might even enjoy watching your partner have sex with someone else. This is what is known as a **cuckold**. Cuck has been misused a lot in recent years to describe someone that treats women like human beings. All a cuckold is, is someone who enjoys the thought of their partner having sex with other people. This can be taken as a submissive or masochist who likes to lose control of their relationship to someone more Dominant, or genuinely enjoys the perceived humiliation of someone else having sex with their partner.

An **exhibitionist** is someone who likes to be watched. An exhibitionist may enjoy undressing in front of their partner or in front of strangers via a webcam. They might enjoy masturbating while others watch or where there is a chance, they might be caught masturbating. Exhibitionists go so far as having sex in front of a crowd like at the Folsom Street Fair.

While there's a good chance you may have heard of all these terms before, if you're a true vanilla, you probably haven't heard of **Gooners**. Gooners are people who participate in vast amounts of edging where they repeatedly masturbate themselves towards orgasm without climaxing. The reasons for this are many. Some people enjoy the control and humiliation of someone deciding if they're allowed to orgasm. Others claim that edging leads to mind shattering orgasms unlike any you could experience from sex. Still others claim to get high off the neurochemicals in their body, similar to a state of being cum drunk.

Know Your Role

After absorbing all this new and exciting information, you're probably wondering where you fit into it. Are you a sub? A sadist? A little even? I can't tell you. I don't know you personally, but I'm sure you're great. The simplest and most effective way to discover where your interests and personality mesh with BDSM is to experiment. You can read a dozen books and watch a hundred people have sex with five-hundred other people, but until you take action, you'll never really know. Start slow, don't try to test everything out in the same night. GO SLOW! Start with mild pain or name calling. Let your partner take control in the bedroom. Use a tie or scarf for some gentle bondage. There's no rush to dive into a role.

As you're experimenting, clear your mind. Try to bring yourself into the moment. Sex isn't about quotas or outside responsibilities. You need to focus on your pleasure and the pleasure of your partner or partners. Sex is about pleasure, freedom, expression, and identity. As stated previously, just because you hold some managerial position doesn't mean you can't be submissive in bed. Just because you're a woman doesn't mean you have to be a masochist or a submissive. If you find you enjoy being Dominant, that doesn't mean you have to go out and buy a leather corset and a crop, though if that makes you feel sexy, go to town.

Don't be ashamed or shocked if you have these notions about what you like during sex then find out it makes you miserable in practice. Remember, 66% of women have fantasized about rape, though virtually none of these women would ever actually want to be forced. Consensual Non-Consent is a thing though and we will discuss it later. You can have all these notions and idea about what it will be like in bed, but until you actually test them, you'll never truly know. Sometimes the reality can never live up to the fantasy you built in your head. Sex isn't about more expectations and responsibilities. Free yourself. Enjoy the things your body responds to, not the things you think you have to respond to.

If you need more help, there is an intensive personality survey you can take online to determine where you fit in the BDSM spectrum. I'm including a link in the footnotes[2]. This is a wonderful, and most importantly, free test you can take to see what suits you. The full test takes less than 10 minutes and you will be asked dozens of questions about your preferred sexual experiences. After the test, you will be given a breakdown of where you fit between Dom and sub, sadist and masochist, etc. If they're willing, have your sexual partner or partners take the test and see where you complement each other. Remember, the results are written in stone. The test is just guide to help you better understand yourself.

Once you determine what aspects of BDSM interest you the most, you must now take the time to determine what kind of dynamic you share with your partner(s). Ideally one of you is a Dominant sadist while the other is a submissive masochist, though in reality, the dynamic rarely breaks down that cleanly. Focus on the aspects of your sexuality that complement each other. No one is obligated to enjoy an aspect of BDSM just because their partner does. In any relationship, you must be willing to make compromises. You can try swapping roles every other occasion or experiment with role reversals. Be accommodating to your partner and ask them to accommodate you. This isn't a competition. No one wins sex. This is about fostering a satisfying sexual relationship.

If worse comes to worse, you can focus on the more vanilla aspects of your sexual relationship. Remember, relationships aren't permanent. You owe it to yourself to preserve your happiness. Compromise can only go so far. I'm not saying you should break up with your partner over sex. You need to decide for yourself how important and intensely satisfying sexual relationship is and if your expectations are realistic. Sometimes sex can ruin a relationship. Sometimes we cling to poor relationships because the sex is fantastic. No one can make these decisions for you. You need to make the decision. You need to talk to your partner or partners if you feel a problem is damaging the relationship.

Psychology Today, *Why Do Women Have Rape Fantasies?* Castleman, Michael, August 2015.
https://www.psychologytoday.com/us/blog/all-about-sex/201508/why-do-women-have-rape-fantasies
https://bdsmtest.org/select-mode

PART II

BDSM IN PRACTICE

♥ ♥ ♥

Now that you have a general understanding of the major parts of BDSM, it's time to put that knowledge into practice. BDSM isn't performed in a book. It's performed in a bedroom, or the shower, or on the kitchen table, or on a pallet in the back of Sam's Club. Uhh... My point is, you know enough about BDSM theory to put it into practice.

Safe

Safe, Sane, and Consensual. Yes, this was already a section in the book. You get a gold star for noticing! (gold stars, available while supplies last). I bring this up again because it is by and far the most important aspect to practicing BDSM. If you're going to learn the ropes (ha, bondage joke) with your favorite partner, then you must always make safety a priority. No act of sex is truly safe, but we can always take steps to minimize harm. Have a general plan in place before you become amorous. I know pre-planned sex is lame, but you don't want to put your partner into a position where they're forced to say no in the heat of things, or are too afraid to say no because they're afraid of how you'll react.

Use plenty of lube. Lube is your friend. Porn gives this really piss poor notion that a horny woman is always dripping and ready to squirt when it often doesn't work like that. Even for vaginal, use lube. There are many kinds of lubes, but the only one I can recommend is generic, water-based lube. There are many kinds of lubes with upsides and downsides. The main downside of water-based lube is it dries out and you need to use more. Other lubes have chemicals like artificial sweeteners and parabens that you don't want anywhere near your genitals. Silicone lube stays slick forever but can degrade sex toys over time. Absolutely under no circumstances should you use Vaseline or petroleum jelly as they'll do serious damage to your insides. I can't recommend oils such as baby oils either as they degrade the latex in condoms and make them unsafe to use. All lubes have their pros and cons, but water-based lube is the only one I'm comfortable recommending.

I know bondage seems exciting and dangerous, and that's because it is. Performing bondage incorrectly can literally lead to death. When bondage is too tight or performed too long, it can create a blood clot. A tiny blood clot can travel to your lungs causing a pulmonary embolism, making it extremely difficult to breath and dangerously lowering the amount of oxygen in your blood to the point of organ failure. A blood clot that travels to the heart can cause a heart attack, and if it travels to the brain, it causes a stroke. This is very unlikely to happen if done correctly. Now that I've thoroughly scared you off from ever attempting bondage, let me explain how to do it safely and effectively.

If you don't want to spend money, you can always use scarves or ties as restraints. The important thing while binding someone's arm and leg is to be able to get two fingers comfortably within the restraint. If you can't, it is too tight and needs to be removed immediately. If you see any discoloration, especially blue or purple skin, or swelling, remove the restraint immediately. If the restraint has been on for several minutes that way, you need to call a paramedic and let them remove the restraint. Removing a restraint that has been on far too long can be deadly. A simply way to remember these rules is to learn your **ABC'S**.

- **A**irways should be unobstructed at all times
- **B**reathing should be gentle and controlled
- **C**irculation should always be maintained
- **S**cissors should be on hands at all times to quickly remove restraints

Gags can be sexy and degrading, but I don't really favor a restraint that blocks your primary airway. If you use a gag, the submissive should be free to remove it at any time. That means not combining a gag with hand restraints.

With or without a gag, breathing should be calm at all times. If you are using a gag, or gagging your partner with your cock, you need to give them time to catch their breath. The last thing you want is someone to be naked and hyper ventilating.

As stated previously, circulation should be maintained at all times. If you feel your limbs becoming tingly, numb, or painfully sensitive, you need to remove your restraints immediately. Scissors should always be close by if a knot cannot be managed.

If you want to graduate beyond homemade restraints, you can shop online for love cuffs. Etsy carries a wide range of sex toys all by small businesses and independent artists. When shopping for cuffs, always purchase soft cuffs made from fabric, or if you choose leather, make sure they have padding. Hard leather cuffs can cut into your skin during sex, and I simply can't recommend anyone use metal cuffs during sex.

I'm sure if you're reading this section you want to learn to tie elaborate and sexy knots. Unfortunately, a book is not the best place to learn such things. There are countless videos on YouTube where you can learn to tie every rope imaginable. With so many knots of varying complexity, it would take an entire book to teach you what you want to know. Fortunately, there is a wonderful website called The Duchy[1] which contains literally hundreds of instructional articles on bondage knot tying.

Sane

While safety addresses the physical wellbeing of all participants, sane attempts to address the mental and emotional aspects of safe sex. Sex is deeply emotional and can trigger all kinds of feelings in us. We can get caught up in the heat of the moment and even do things we later regret. The most important thing is to enter any sexual situation of sound mind and body. I know drinking or smoking weed is a great way to relax and destroy some inhibitions, but you shouldn't be so high or intoxicated to the point you don't remember what happened the night before. You always want to be in your complete faculties so you maintain control of the situation. You should never be pressured into a sexual situation if you feel you are too intoxicated. It is absolutely okay to refuse sex, even if the request/demand is from your spouse or partner. It is never okay to pressure someone, guilt someone, or beg someone for sex. That is despicable behavior.

If you are extremely angry or depressed, sex might not be the best thing for you. It's okay to use sex to cheer yourself up, but you shouldn't enter a sexual situation where you might hurt someone out of anger or allow your Dom to take things too far because you are feeling worthless. Sex is about freedom and pleasure; it should never be about punishing yourself or others because of your unchecked emotions.

On the opposite end of the spectrum, sometimes it can be difficult for a person to hurt their partner during sex. You love and cherish this person and never want to cause them pain. First, you should never force your partner to hurt you if it causes them emotional distress. Second, at least make an attempt to satisfy the masochist needs of your partner. You're just hurting them, not harming them. Think about shiatsu massage or spicy food. These two things objectively hurt, but their ultimate goal is pleasure and millions of people enjoy them. Don't think you're protecting your partner by refusing to engage their masochistic desires. You honor and respect your partner by giving them the agency to make that decision, not by deciding you know better than them. Try hurting them at least once if they desire so. If they hate it, you truly know them better than they know themselves. But if they enjoy it, you have entered a new level of intimacy with them. Masochism, like sex, is a very intimate act we only share with a few people on our lifetimes. Your partner loves and trusts you so much they want you to hurt them knowing that you care about their wellbeing and will stop when they tell you to. That is a serious level of intimacy.

I'd like to finish this section by discussing a little understood phenomenon known as being cum drunk, sometimes called cock drunk. There are times during a sexual encounter when the foreplay and/or sex is so incredible that it feels like you are high or drunk. Everything is clicking, your body is responding, and you feel like the porn star you were born to be. This feeling can reach dizzying heights to the point you no longer feel like you're in control anymore. You can feel like a raving whore an animal in heat. This is what is known as being cum drunk. There's not enough research on this esoteric phenomenon, but I have been with partners and read interviews with sex workers who claim to have gone through this. From what I've been told, cum drunk is an incredible thing. It's this state where your inhibitions are completely eroded away and you simply become sex. Trust me when I say it leads to the most amazing sexual experiences of your life. The important thing to try and remember when you or your partner is cum drunk is to not do anything you will regret or have lasting consequences. Cum drunk people might want to toss condoms out the window and take cock raw, but there are serious consequences for doing so. You may want to attempt risky or taboo things like having sex in public or taking naughty photos. I know such things can be intensely erotic and fuel your cum drunk state in the moment, but it's important to keep some grasp on common sense. It may be up to you or your partner to keep things sane as it were while the other persons rides the flood of hormones and neurotransmitters.

Consent

Arguably the most important aspect of all BDSM is consent. While I don't really believe any of the aspects of BDSM or safe, sane, consensual should be weighed against each other, without consent, there is nothing. Make no mistake, I don't care what the circumstances are, a person can withdraw consent at any time for any reason or no reason at all. If you do not honor lack of consent, you have no respect for your partner as a human being and shouldn't even be allowed to be in a room with them, let alone a relationship.

When it comes to things like Domination and submission, consent can become blurry if you do not plan ahead. This is why limits and safe-words are so important. I know we discussed them in a previous chapter, but they're so critical to a safe and positive BDSM experience, I would like to reiterate and expand upon them. Plus, I don't want to assume every person is reading the chapters in chronological order. Limits are actions or behaviors that are forbidden during sex. A Dominant and submissive can both have their own limits and they must always be honored. Like pretzels, there are two kinds of limits, soft and hard. Soft limits are actions that can be broken under special circumstances, usually when a submissive is intensely aroused and craving me taboo or depraved things. When a submissive is cum drunk, soft limits are frequently broken as inhibitions become shattered. It's okay to test your partner's soft limits, but you must respect when they refuse or tell you to stop. Hard limits are limits that are not allowed to be broken under any circumstances. Even in the heat of the moment when your submissive is cum drunk and begging for a hard limit to be broken, you must honor your prior commitment. If they truly wanted their limit broken, they should have designated it as a soft limit beforehand. The entire point of limits is to respect you and your partner's agency and dignity.

If your limits are nebulous or you don't have enough experience to know everything you like and dislike, safe-words are a failsafe. I don't care what the circumstance is, it is never okay to press on when someone utters their safe-word. A safe-word brings all sexual activity to a halt until the person who uttered it decides if and when they want to continue. In my eyes, willfully failing to acknowledge a safe-word is the same as rape. A safe-word should be a word that would never be uttered in the course of sexual activity. "No" and "Stop" are atrocious safe-words as sometimes a submissive can enjoy uttering those words in a playful or teasing manner to heighten the experience. Foods, months, and seasons are simple and easy to remember safe-words. It doesn't hurt to write it down and put a post-it up if you're just starting out. If your partner starts yelling strange words, chances are they forgot what the safe-word is and are trying to make you stop. If speech is not possible, whether you or your partner are deaf, or your mouth is gagged, safe actions can also be used. A bell to ring, something unusual that is obvious during the course of amorous activity, like throwing up a peace sign. There should be no mistake when someone is trying to pause the action.

Before we can close this section on consent, we must talk about a specific kink called consensual non-consent. Consensual non-consent is where two or more people roleplay a rape or forced sex. When engaging in this type of roleplay, safety should always be the first order of business. Roleplaying such a violent scenario is fraught with pitfalls, especially when bondage is brought into the mix. There are many ways to participate in consensual non-consent, but only one way to do it safely. Bear in mind I've only ever read about this happening where women pretend to be the rape victim during a roleplay, though it is full possibly for a man to play the role, regardless of the gender of their partner. In some scenarios, the rape victim is abducted by the rapist, brought somewhere secluded, usually their own bedroom, and the two engage in sex. How violent, and degrading the sex is, and how much bondage is involved, should be discussed beforehand, though some rape victims prefer not to know when they'll be kidnaped or how they'll be raped.

Basically, in consensual non-con, there is a pull between making the sex as safe as possible, and the roleplay as realistic as possible. As a sex educator, I can only advise that you take every reasonable safety precaution possible. If abduction is part of the roleplay, don't do it in public where a bystander could mistake your roleplay for a real felony. Plan the roleplay around your own homes. The rape victim can simply enter their home and be jumped by their assailant. Sometimes the victim doesn't want to know what is going to happen to them. Again, I can only advise that you plan beforehand and give clear limits as well as a safe-word. It's not uncommon for the victim in the roleplay to forsake the use of a safe-word to make the rape as realistic as possible. I cannot disagree with this more. There must always be a failsafe in any sexual situation. I know the thought of the guy or girl not stopping no matter what is an insane turn on and simulates actual rape, but it's dangerous. You can end up serious hurt or forced into an act you hate and/or causes several pain or distress. Sometimes a roleplay victim will recruit a stranger from the internet to play the assailant. Again, I cannot recommend this. Consensual non-consent is so fraught with peril that you should only really do it with someone you trust. I know all these rules seem like a bummer and a total turn-off, but it would be irresponsible of me to not stress every measure you can take to preserve your health and dignity.

To the Victims of Sexual Abuse

I don't know where to put this caveat, but I figure after the section on consent would be the best place. I talk about this often with other BDSM practitioner and feel it deserves its own attention. Rape and sexual abuse plague our society. Many of us have to live our daily lives knowing we had serious emotional and physical violence done to us. Some of us overcome and move on while others battle every day to cope. You are not an inferior or damaged person because you were assaulted. You weren't drawn to BDSM because some part of you is broken or twisted. It's quite possible that you were drawn to BDSM because you wish to regain control of your sexuality instead of letting a crime dictate how you should feel towards sex.

There is nothing wrong with a sexual assault victim who engages in any aspect of BDSM. BDSM is simply an umbrella term that breaks down most kinks and fetishes into their paradigms. You are not suddenly more perverted because you want to be a more sexual person. Just because you were raped or molested doesn't meant you're not allowed to enjoy submission, bondage, or masochism. You're not broken. You are taking control of your sexuality. You are defining your sexuality on your own terms. I have spoken with too many survivors of sexual assault, and when appropriate, I have found that many, not all but many, of them either masturbate to their assault or fantasize about something similar happening again. I want to tell you right now that is perfectly normal and healthy. You are taking this violent and degrading act that was forced upon you, and deciding how it makes you feel. You are taking the guilt and shame and turning it into a beautiful and pleasurable orgasm. Don't let that act of violence that was done to you dictate your sex live going forward. Follow the rules of safe, sane, and consensual, and decide for yourself what makes you aroused.

Start Creating a Scene

One of the best parts of BDSM is the ability to create scenes that you and your partner(s) roleplay. While roleplaying isn't for everyone, I'm creating this section under the presumption that you either love roleplaying your fantasies, want to try it, and/or want to get better at it. Since BDSM largely encompasses all aspects of the sexual experience, you can take the pieces and parts you want to create exciting and kinky scenarios. Want to be the naughty student kept after class by your teacher? Maybe some Domination and submission is involved. There's no reason you can't toss some spanking into the scenario as well.

Some people just aren't great at roleplaying or can't get into the headspace. You're effectively acting, and not everyone is an actor. To immerse yourself in a scene, it can certainly help to use costumes or props. Sure, you can pretend your girlfriend is a cop, but what if she's wearing a uniform, has a baton, and big aviator sunglasses? Want your boyfriend to be a prisoner that ravages your body? Have him get a henna tattoo and an orange jumpsuit. Wigs are excellent and affordable for roleplaying because it can make you feel like you're having sex with a completely different person. Don't downplay the effectiveness of lingerie in the bedroom. Some people have a response to lingerie where it feels like they're being given permission to act more sexual and sluttier.

When roleplaying, it certainly helps to be openminded. Don't dismiss your partner's fantasies out of hand because they don't immediately appeal to you. Sexual experimentation is critical to finding the things that turn you on the most. Maybe you think your partner's school teacher fantasy is lame, but you play along and suddenly you find out you enjoy Dominating and spanking them.

Don't be afraid to break the rules. Roleplay is where you have permission to be whoever you want. You can pretend to be someone underage or even pretend to be one of your relatives of one of your partner's relatives. It's just roleplaying between two consenting adults. You're not hurting anyone. These are just fantasies. You wouldn't get mad at your partner because they shot a bunch of people in a videogame, would you? Roleplaying is just another fantasy.

If you need ideas, don't be afraid to draw from movies, TV shows, books, or even videogames. Maybe your boyfriend has a thing for Lara Croft? Maybe your girlfriend has a thing for Jon Snow? The possibilities are literally endless. If you've been getting bored of the same sexual experience every week, then roleplaying is the perfect opportunity to spice things up for the rest of your life.

It might help if you and your partner keep lists of scenes you want to try or fictional characters you want to have sex with. Don't be afraid to fill a notebook with ideas and show them to your partner. For all you know, the both of you have similar scenes you want to try. Porn can be an inspiration too, but I find the most satisfying roleplays come from our own imagination.

Sex Toys and Accessories

I believe one of the simplest and most effective ways to spice up your sex life is to incorporate toys in the bedroom. No, I'm not talking about Legos, and Play-Doh, though they're both awesome and inspire creativity, I'm talking about sex toys. Etsy is the ideal place for hand crafted sex toys where you can support small businesses and artists. For more complicated sex toys, Amazon is your best bet. If you find Amazon morally objectionable, you can try Adam and Eve, Spencer's Gifts, or your local adult shop though the prices won't always be competitive. We have a lot to get through, so let's start where it all began.

When people think of sex toys, they usually think of the humble **dildo**. A dildo is usually just a silicone cock. It's really that simple, I don't know what revelations you were expecting me to bring. Well...there are a few things I can teach you. The difference between a dildo and a vibrator is that a vibrator vibrates, though vibrators are often called dildos. You know you can soak a dildo in warm water to make it comfortably warm like it's an actual cock? You can also use a condom with your dildo to make clean up much simpler. When it comes to cleaning a dildo, warm soapy water is usually enough. Some people sanitize them in their dishwasher. I recommend you use the top rack so you don't melt the dildo. Silicone dildo's come in a variety of firmness's and it's important you find the one most comfortable for you. Glass dildos are safer than they sound as glass actually has incredible tensile strength. Glass dildos tend to be unpleasantly firm and need to be warmed up before use though. Some dildos have two heads and are designed to be used be a lesbian couple genital to genital for double penetration. Never, ever use silicone lube with a silicone dildo as the lube can make the dildo feel tacky and unpleasant after washing. As far as **strap-on's** go, they're just harnesses a dildo can be slid into to double as a penis.

There are many kinds of dildos besides basic ones that look like penises. That are special dildos called prostate stimulators designed especially for men. While men can derive great satisfaction from the use of a dildo, prostate stimulators are designed especially for men and especially for solo use as dildoing your own butt requires some degree of flexibility to avoid muscle cramps. Dildoing your butt is safe for both men and women who can derive great degrees of pleasure from anal stimulation. Make sure to use plenty of lube and to go slow. Your asshole has thousands of tender nerve endings.

In addition to dildos, **butt-plugs** are another similar toy designed exclusive for your bum. They are very similar to a dildo though generally only a couple inches in length and a flared based. The flared base is designed to stop your anus from swallowing the plug which usually requires a doctor to have removed because of the physics of your anus. I highly recommend using butt plugs with only the widest bases to prevent such an embarrassing situation. On Amazon you can find many sets of butt plugs that come in small-medium-large sizes to train up your tolerance for anal. Some butt plugs have a jewel in them. These are called princess plugs and the jewel is visible when the plug is in your asshole. There are also butt plugs with animal tails attached. The most common are horses and ferrets for god knows what reason. There are also curly pig tails and tails from My Little Pony. Don't worry, I left a link to the My Little Pony butt plug in the foot notes[2] so you can see for yourself.

Aside from the generic dildo and butt plugs, there are also dildos designed to resemble the cocks of animals. The most common are dog and horse dildos, though Bad Dragon[3] has a vast array of artisan dildos designed to look like the cocks of mythical creatures. Aside from their interesting business model, I'd like to point out that Bad Dragon dildos are made to order and are completely customizable. You can dictate the size and firmness of the dildo as well as the color scheme. You can also decide if your dildo has a suction base and/or shoots cum lube which is milky white lube that looks like cum. They have won many awards for the quality of their sex toys and have inspired a loyal following in the BDSM community.

Vibrators are the energetic sisters of dildos, and you can quote me on that. Vibrators vibrate and dildos generally don't, though there are dildos with a pocket you can insert a vibrating bullet in to turn it into dildo. There are metal and silicone vibrators. Some vibrators strongly resemble cocks while other vibrators resemble personal massagers and tend to be much more powerful. While all vibrators vibrate, others have several functions. Some vibrators can gyrate to simulate the strokes and swirls of an actual cock. Others have a rabbit attachment that stimulates the clit directly. Rabbits are tiny vibrators you can wear on your finger and stimulate your clit specifically. Despite popular belief, your clit will not become desensitized with constant use of a rabbit or vibrator. Any numbness you feel after a vibration orgasm is only temporary. Do not be afraid to go to town and rely on your vibrator for all your orgasms. There are also vibrating bullets and vibrating eggs that are exactly what they sound like. I don't know what would happen if you shot someone with a vibrating bullet, but if you slip it inside you it can feel amazing. These special toys usually have a controller to control how hard they vibrate. Some bullets and eggs have a special controller that interfaces with your cellphone or music player and vibrates to the bass line. With modern technology, we also have eggs and bullets that can be controlled wirelessly with a smartphone app or wireless controller. You can send orgasms to your partner from literally thousands of miles away.

Besides the toys that penetrate, there are also toys that can be penetrated. These toys have a lot of names, the most common being called **stroker's, masturbators, pocket pussies, and fleshlights**. They all generally mean the same thing, a silicone orifice that can be repeatedly penetrated for pleasure. They come in tons of different sizes, makes and qualities. Almost all of them are designed to resemble a pussy, mouth, or asshole. The insides are textures to increase pleasure stimulation. As far as recommendations go, you get what you pay for. Cheap stroker's can feel like literally fucking plastic while expensive ones feel shockingly like the real thing. You can go on Bad Dragon and find stroker's modeled after the orifices of fantasy creatures. Fleshlight has a series of stroker's cast from the actual vaginas of famous porn stars so it feels like you're actually fucking them. I don't know how you know if they were true to form though. Would you be fucking the Riley Reid one when suddenly you realize you're in Dominika Butterfly's pussy and call up to demand a refund? Some stroker's are actual silicone butts you can penetrate, while others go all the way and give you a limbless torso to fondle and fuck. All in all, stroker's are amazing and will completely change the quality of your orgasms for the better. It's really one of the best investments you can make into the quality of your life.

You may be surprised to learn that a wide arrays clamps and accessories exist for all your needs. As mentioned before, if you do not want to purchases nipple clamps you can use clothespin, stay fresh chip clips, pliers, or an adjustable wrench. If you are shopping for nipple clamps, I highly recommend you begin with adjustable alligator clamps. These alligator clamps will typically be linked by a chain and the teeth will be covered with a rubber or silicone grip. Please don't remove the cover of the teeth. Behind the teeth is a bolt that controls how tightly the clamps close. This is perfect for those new to pain or nipple play. Some nipple clamps have no chain but instead bells or tassels on the end for aesthetic pleasure. Some even vibrate though cheap vibrating ones tend to slip off. In addition to alligator clamps there are also clover clamps. Clover clamps resemble a tiny pair of pliers and can be very painful if you're not used to nipple torture. Tweezer clamps look just like a pair of tweezers with rubber tips. A metal ring slides down the length of the tweezer clamps to control pressure. Finally, there is something called a nipple press where a ring circles your nipple and rounded bolts are twisted in until it pinches your nipple. Bear in mind all the clamps listed typically have versions with aesthetic accessories attached as well as vibrating options to heighten pleasure. While not technically a clamp, nipple suckers are small tubes you attach to your nipples and create suction, temporarily distending your nipples. This is largely painless and the intent is to heighten sensitivity and have more nipple to work with in case you have small nipples. When attaching clamps, you generally want to the mouth to pinch the areola behind the nipple so the clamp remained attached during sex. A word of warning, after a while, your nipples go numb from using clamps, but taking the clamp off is extremely painful if the clamp has been on awhile.

For the sake of posterity, we will also discuss **cock rings and cock cages**. The thing about cock cages, also known as male chastity belts, is you either love them or think they're weird. It's important not to judge others for their sexual preferences. What you might think is weird might be an insane turn on for someone else. Something that makes you horny might be totally off-putting to another person. A cock cage is made from plastic or metal and is worn over the penis to prevent erections. When fitted properly, the cage around the penis will prevent any meaningful erections. To measure your penis for a cage or ring, the easiest thing to do is wrap a strip of paper around your flaccid penis and use that to measure the circumference. Divide that number by 3.14 and you have your diameter. With the diameter, you can fit yourself to any device you see fit. A cock ring is very similar to a chastity belt, minus the cage. It is proven that with a cock ring in place you will have harder erections that last longer and reduce the chance of premature ejaculation. Size is everything though. A ring that is too tight can cause injury, and if the ring is too lose it won't work. Don't be afraid to use a little lube getting the ring or cage on. A cock ring should not be worn for longer than 30 minutes at a time while technically a cock cage can be worn a week at a time. I cannot recommend more than 2 days followed by a good scrubbing. All of us have dirty, dirty, genitals that need to be washed regularly. If a cock cage is too tight, it can break the skin then cause an infection. Like nipple clamps, there are cock rings that vibrate, though this is actually designed for the pleasure of your female part as the vibrations press against her clit. Though spiked male chastity belts exist, I cannot in good conscience recommend anyone use them out of fear of broken skin.

I feel like I covered cuffs enough in the safety section, but **rope** bondage is also hugely popular in the BDSM community. All the safety tips you learned still apply when attempting rope bondage. Like lube, there are many kinds of bondage rope, each with their own pros and cons. For a beginner I highly recommend cotton rope. It feels good against your skin and it's very cheap. The main problem is that knots can get stuck if pulled too tight. Polypropylene rope is also common and inexpensive, but the rope doesn't have very good bite, meaning knots tend to come undone. Nylon rope is the kind of general-purpose white rope or yellow rope used in construction and boating. While it is more expensive than cotton rope, it will last much longer, but some knots simply won't stay with nylon. Hemp is popular with aesthetic rope binding in America. Hemp can feel unpleasant against your skin and you'll need to pay more for smooth hemp rope. The last type of bondage rope I want to talk about is jute. Jute rope is made from a special plant fiber called jute (duh). It is much more expensive than cotton but certainly not outside of most people's price range. If you are serious about some expert level rope bondage, jute is where it's at.

I'll close this massive section with a word about **porn and erotica**. BDSM and toys give us the instructions and means for a fun and safe sexual experience, but it is often tasty smut that inspires us to try new and interesting things. Whether you prefer the written word, pictures, homemade movies, or professionally made videos, there is porn out there for you. Speaking to the women specifically, I know it can feel like porn isn't designed for you, and the truth is, it isn't. Porn is made by men and for men. The industry argues that women just don't view as much porn as men. While that is true, it fails to take into account the reality that they're not catering to female audiences. It is also true women read more porn than men. Regardless of how you prefer to consume your erotic content, there are many options for you. For basic free porn, Pornhub[4] and XVideos[5] are the hands down the most popular free porn sites on the internet as of the writing of this book. They are generally virus free and contain millions of free videos in addition to useful search features and category options. If you prefer still images or animated gifs that allow your imagination to run wild, Sex.com contains an excellent selection of images and animated gifs sorted into helpful categories. It's true you can find porn just about anywhere, but you should only ever use trusted and recommended sites as many, MANY porn sites contain viruses and malware. If you want a premium BDSM experience, then Kink.com is the last stop you'll ever need to make. Kink.com is actually 70 different sites in one, and you'll have access to all of them with a single subscription. They're based out of San Francisco, are known for their diverse hiring practices, giving back to the community, their healthy and safe work environment, as well as firing James Dean immediately after accusations came out. If you prefer written smut, then Literotica[6] is your last stop for unlimited free erotica. While the site can be difficult to navigate, you won't find a larger collection of free erotica anywhere else on the internet.

Impact Play

I've separated Impact play from the rest of the toys because there is quite a bit of safety and precaution that needs to be taken as well as addressing the various toys that go along with it. Impact play is when you strike your partner for one or both of your sexual pleasure. this can be done simply with the hand across the chest or butt, but it can be so much more elaborate than that. Before I discuss the toys and methods, I want to take a moment to discuss the **stoplight method**. The stoplight method is a simple set of commands you can use when engaging with impact play with your partner or partners. During impact play, you can say **green** which means everything is fine or you want your partner to increase the pain or rhythm of the impact. If you say **yellow**, that means you are approaching your pain threshold and your partner needs to slow down or maintain their current intensity. **Red** means things have gone too far and you need to stop immediately. When performing impact play, the safest plays to play are the butt and chest. I do not advise striking the back or lower torso as this can cause muscle pain, bruised ribs, or in the worst-case scenario, organ damage. A firm strike to the liver can leave your partner momentarily paralyzed with pain. Aside from the flat of your hand, there are many, many toys used for impact play and I'm going to attempt to name them all for you. The one I bet you're expecting most is the classic whip. This is actually a pretty rare BDSM toy. You certainly won't see whips that are several feet long like you do in TV and in movies. A real BDSM whip is around 52 inches and made from leather. Similar to a whip is what is known as a flogger. A flogger has a small handle with several strips of leather attached to it resembling a mop head. Floggers are a great beginning tool because light flogging actually feels very comfortable and you have the control to ramp up the impact later on. Similar to a flogger is the humble crop. A flogger is a flexible cane with flat tip made of leather. Crops are also excellent beginner's toys as the light weight and flat head allow you to easily control how much pain you deliver. Rods and canes are also used in BDSM but I don't really recommend them. Typically, they're not graded for use on people for impact play. Rods can break and canes can cause injury. Paddles are another fun tool, though I highly recommend a flexible leather paddle that allows you to control how much force you deliver instead of a stiff wooden paddle that can cause injury.

As far as safety goes, remember the stoplight method. If an area of the body is becoming crimson, take a break and allow the tissue to recover. Even light impact play done repeatedly can cause broken skin. If you have bloody redness on the site of impact that looks like a rash, that's actually broken skin. Don't hesitate to rub Vaseline or bacitracin on the broken skin to prevent infection.

Aftercare

No discussion of BDSM would be complete without discussing aftercare. Aftercare is the post-coital ritual of tending to your partner's physical, mental, and emotional needs. Sex is an intensely emotional experience and can become much more intense as you explore the depths of your kinks and fantasies. BDSM taps into a subconscious, lower brain part of our psyche. When we engage without most desired kinks, the results can be explosive. Many people have compared a quality BDSM session to a religious experience, and I would have to agree with them. When the mood is right, you and your partner(s) are clicking, and all the bases are covered, it can feel like you are ascending to another level of reality. You're set for the best sex of your life after reading this book. You have all the tools and knowledge you need to become cum drunk. If you've never had a quality sexual experience you may be asexual, or there's a good possibility you've never been with a competent partner. Good sex will change who you are on a fundamental level. You will experience the highest of highs, but that also means that the lowest of lows can follow.

Masochist's and submissive's are prime candidates for aftercare, though anyone of any role can require it after sex. Aftercare is the time to hit pause or stop and tend to the non-sexual needs of your partner. If you have been through an intense sadomasochism session, now is the time to tend to the physical and emotional wounds of your partner. Remember, during intense arousal all kinds of hormones and neurotransmitters are surging through your body. Over a long enough period of time, you can literally get high on your own bodily chemicals. But all highs have a crash. Some people cope better than others. Even if your sub often insists, they don't need aftercare, always offer it just to keep their best interests at heart. If dealing with a masochist, make sure where you struck them or tortured them is free from broken skin. If necessary, tend to any wounds you accidentally inflicted. Remember, this isn't just about tending to their physical damage. Hold them and comfort them. Let them know they are loved and cared for. If you verbally berated them or insulted them, reassure them that you didn't mean the things you said.

Some submissive require a lot of time and attention after sex. Plan your night accordingly. It is absolutely your responsibility to tend to the emotional needs of your submissive after sex. Even if your session involved no sadomasochism, embodying the role of a submissive can take tremendous courage and energy. They are giving up control to you. Think about how difficult it would be to give up control of your life to another person. There is a considerable emotional component to submitting and you must honor their sacrifice. Some subs need to be held and comforted after sex. Others need their space. Don't be afraid to wrap them in a blanket like a big burrito. If the session has gone for hours (yes, with BDSM you can have mind-blowing sex for literal hours if you pace yourself), your partner might require food and drink. Don't hesitate to make their favorite food or snack and give them time to come down. Put on their favorite show and tend to their needs. If you are dealing with a little, have their favorite stuffed animal nearby to snuggle.

Once you practice BDSM enough, you'll understand how intense it can be. Whether you are a sadist or a masochist, a Dom or a sub, it's okay to ask for aftercare. You're not imposing on your partner by suddenly becoming emotionally needy. If you both need aftercare at the same time, this is the perfect chance to bond and create intimacy. You can just lay in bed for hours and share each other's embrace and hour takeout. BDSM is about freedom and pleasure. You are nurturing a side of yourself that has been neglected for years. It can be really intense. Don't be ashamed if you cry or become emotional. Just perform your duty as a loving and caring sexual partner. Be the kind of sexual partner you would want to be with when it comes to aftercare. And remember, not everyone needs aftercare. We all process emotions differently. Some people won't have the same emotional response as you. Just because your partner doesn't become intensely emotional after sex, doesn't mean they didn't have an amazing time. Communicate with each other. It's such a stupid notion that two people exchanging sexual fluids think it's awkward to discuss what they want before, during, or after sex. Tell your partner how the experience made you feel. Tell them what they could do differently next time or let them know something you want to try in the future. But don't forget to praise them for the things they did right.

I think people want to be in the kind of relationship where they don't have to communicate their needs to each other. They want to be in the kind of relationship where they're so in tune with one another, it's almost like a psychic connection. Well I have to say, that's a great way to not get your needs met ever. Don't assume your partner knows what you like and don't like. TELL YOUR PARTNER WHAT YOU LIKE AND DON'T LIKE. This isn't a time for secrets or meaningful looks. BDSM is about, freedom, pleasure, and expression. Now is the best time to convey your emotional needs to your partner. If you both can do that, I guarantee you'll grow closer as a couple.

PART III

WHERE DO I START?

♥ ♥ ♥

S o, you know the theory and methods behind BDSM. You know what it means, you know what to expect, you understand the safety precautions to take for a fun and pleasant experience. All that's left to do is start. But where do you start? BDSM contains a dizzying array of activities, each one with its own appeal. The most important thing you can do is start by communicating. Communication will be constantly emphasized in this chapter and for good reason. Communication is key to any successful relationship. Things start to fall apart when you stop communicating. If you are afraid or reluctant to tell your partner how you feel, then the relationship is already suffering. How you communicate is arguably more important than the things you actually say.

If you want to incorporate BDSM into your relationship, don't start by saying you find your sex life deeply miserable and unsatisfied. That immediately puts your partner on the defensive. Instead mention how you picked up this book and found a lot of kinky ideas you want to try out. The best thing you can do is share this book with your partner or partners so you're all on the same page. This is an excellent strategy because then you don't have to explain to your partner all the roles, rules, and dynamics of BDSM. They'll also have a chance to find inspiration for the things they might want to try.

This isn't about convincing them your sex life is broken or anything. Think of it this way. Imagine if your partner made buttered noodles every night. You may love buttered noodles, and your partner might even make them well, but there's nothing wrong with wanting to try other food besides buttered noodles. You certainly don't have to practice BDSM every night or even every time you have sex. The best thing you can do is take things nice and slow.

Calm, intelligent people can turn into frightened woodland creatures when it comes to sex. The most confident and outgoing person can wither when you want to discuss sex with them and how to improve it. The worst scenario is when your partner thinks you have an amazing sex life when in reality you are less than satisfied with it. Go nice and slow, like.

Your First BDSM Session

If you ever played Pokémon, your first BDSM session is like trying to catch an Abra. One wrong move and they'll teleport away. This is especially true if your partner is overconfident in their sexual prowess. Go slow. The most basic thing you can do to avoid a disaster is to forego anything particularly painful. Focus on dirty talk, light bondage, and light roleplay. Don't be afraid to call your partner mommy or daddy. Some people really respond to that kind of dirty talk. Don't try to over analyze what it implies, just be in the moment. Call your partner sir or ma'am if you're feeling submissive. If you're feeling bolder, discuss beforehand if your partner wants to do some dirty talk. Don't be afraid to toss around terms like slut or stud. Dirty talk can be a minefield, so it's important you go nice and slow. Start with the light stuff and get feedback from your partner. If they're enthused, move onto dirtier. Pace yourself. Do not bury them in an avalanche of insults. Less is more when it comes to dirty talk. Often guys see a girl respond to name-calling during sex and just bury them in a rap battle's worth of insults. If slut works out for you, try bitch, whore, cunt. Spread this out over more than one session. If your partner is truly feeling the verbal abuse, try calling them a pig, cow, cocksleeve. You may just discover that your partner has a huge masochistic side they didn't even know about. People change during the heat of sex. Inhibitions shatter, boundaries are erased. Learn about your partner. Be receptive to your needs.

If verbal abuse feels too risky, then begin with light bondage. The simplest thing you can do to spice up your sex life is to add a blindfold. With your partner blindfolded, go nice and slow. Have them sit on the bed fully clothed and blindfold themselves. Slowly enter the room. Move around. Make some noise. Go through some drawers as if you are searching for something. Start by undressing them. Go nice and slow. Their primary sense is completely cut off. The blindfold will make them feel helpless as you have your way with them. Touch them. Touch their nipples, their lips, their genitals. Stroke them everywhere. Go down on them. Pleasure your partner. With the blindfold on, you'll have to guide them through every action. Have them perform oral sex on you. You are in complete control as they pleasure you. If afterwards your partner enjoyed going down on you blindfolded, there is an excellent chance they are submissive. With just a blindfold you have created an intense BDSM experience.

If the blindfold was a success, I urge you to consider love cuffs for your next sexual adventure. There is just something about being put into restraints during sex that completely opens up your body to pleasure. There is this feeling of helplessness like you are just at the mercy of your partner. I'm leaving a link in the notes for a pair of cute, affordable, and easy to remove sex cuffs[1]. If you still feel uncomfortable buying sex toys (really, still?) you can use a scarf, neck tie, or bandana. Just having your hands bound in front of you can make sex take on a completely different feeling. I would absolutely not start with tying someone to the bed. Some people can feel panicked or claustrophobic when they're restrained. Always start simple and build up over multiple sessions. Start with hands in front of the back, then maybe behind the back, then maybe face up on the bed with hands tied above your head. There is no rush. If you're dealing with a vanilla partner like yourself, the imperative is to go slow and make them aroused but comfortable.

Another simple peace of bondage that can have explosive results in the bedroom is a sex collar. While a collar doesn't necessarily surrender control to the other person, some people feel like it gives them permission to be kinky. Submissives use it to signal that they are ready to be submissive sexually. With a leash attached, you can actually control the other person. Make sure you use a leash and collar designed for human use and not for dogs. Sex collars are cushions so they don't chafe against the neck. Treat your partner like you would your pet. Have them sit in your lap or kneel for you. Absolutely do not yank on the collar or you can injure them.

Don't be afraid to put on the blindfold, cuffs, or leash yourself. Don't go into BDSM assuming you already know everything you like and don't like. This is a time for freedom and experimentation. Your gender cannot dictate what you find erotic. You and your partner(s) are in this together. There's no shame in discovering you are submissive or a masochist.

If bondage feels too risky for your vanilla lover, feel free to incorporate a toy. Full stop, you will have a tremendous amount of difficulty convincing your straight male partner to put something in his butt. For this recommendation, the focus is using a toy on you, your female partner, or your highly willing male partner. If you've never bought a dildo or vibrator before that's absolutely fine, though I think after using one you will find you have been doing yourself a great disservice to yourself all these years. Start small. There is no hurry to buy a great big swinging dildo that can be used for home defense. While Etsy is a great resource for handmade and unique dildos, Amazon sells quality dildos dirt cheap. I'm including a link in the footnotes for a decent started dildo that only costs $10 at the time of this writing[2]. Now more than ever, it is imperative that you go slow and gentle. Whether you are using this on yourself or your partner, don't go with the expectation the pussy will be soaking wet and ready to swallow the entire toy. The vagina expands and contracts based on a number of circumstances. Use as much water-based lube as you want. Spit is not a suitable lubricant for sex. If this toy is going in someone's butt, all care and concern must be exhibited. If you push an asshole too far, they will push back with a vengeance. The butthole is so freaking sensitive. It's literally a guy's g-spot. And yes, guys can cum from prostate stimulation alone. Be gentle, use plenty of lube. Wash your toys after every use. If you want to get started on the butt path, I've included a link for an anal starter set[3]. I think you'll be pleasantly surprised at how intensely erotic it is to masturbate your partner.

Whether or not you found name-calling, blindfolds, or toys to your liking, the next step is to incorporate some gentle yet rough pain in your lovemaking. I know it can be fun and exciting to incorporate surprises into sex, but I truly believe the best sex has a plan and expectations. Sex shouldn't be high risk, high reward. This is an intimate setting. Don't scare or offend your partner by pulling aggressive sex out of nowhere. Before you begin light pain, I strongly advise you to sit down with your partner or partners and tell them you want to try things a little rough next time. I've said it a thousand times, GO SLOW. The simplest and least risky thing you can do is start with some spanking. If you've never spanked your partner before start gentle. Give them a light slap on the butt and tell them how bad they've been. If they respond well, you can be firmer. If the spanking is going very well, I highly

71

recommend you incorporate a flogger into your lovemaking. A flogger is more like a tool for massage than a tool for pain, though without enough force, anything is painful. Start gently with the flogger. You'll soon realize that being gently flogged actually feels like a massage. If you or your partner is being naughty, a firm swat of the butt is usually enough to sort them out.

If spanking goes well, try to incorporate biting during sex. Be very gentle during biting. You don't need to chomp down on someone. Often, it's not even about causing pain. Just the pressure of the bite and possessiveness it implies is enough to around your partner. You can bite your partner's toes, nipples, arms, shoulders, butt, or ears. The ears are an excellent place to nibble. Just a little pressure as you exhale on their neck and shoulder, awakening their erogenous zone.

Hair pulling is a sexy way to incorporate BDSM in the bedroom, but you must do it responsibly. Hair pulling is idea with a longhaired partner. Grab a good fistful of hair away from the root and just hold them. Absolutely do not yank their head back or jerk them side to side. Hair pulling can feel very intense, especial during doggy style as you effectively ride them.

Face slapping is risky, but some people respond it to very well. Less is more when it comes to the face. Always use the flat of your hand against the meat of their cheek.

The Stoplight System

I know we discussed the stoplight system previously, but it is truly ideal for those new to BDSM, not just for those who do impact play. Basically, whenever you are trying anything new or risky in the bedroom, the stoplight system is perfect for a positive experience. When things are calm and comfortable and need to be escalated, you say green. Like a traffic light, green is the signal to keep going. If things are going too fast or you don't want them to escalate further, you say yellow. Just like in traffic, the yellow light means to be cautious and slow down. Red means stop. Red always means stop. If your partner says red, then it's time to take a break. Maybe the sex is becoming too painful, or they're just not feeling it tonight. Maybe you pushed your limits too far. Your partner doesn't need a specific reason to say red, all you have do is respect them.

When you combine the stoplight system with a safe-word, soft limits, hard limits, an open mind and adventurous spirit, you are guaranteed to experience better sex. It's all about communication. Plenty of planning and communication leads to a better sexual experience, but also communicating in the heat of the moment will prevent any serious disasters or hurt feelings. Sex isn't designed for you to lay there and endure misery while your partner gets off. It should be about mutual pleasure. If one of you orgasms every time and the other person is miserable, THAT'S NOT NORMAL. That's crappy sex and you should never have to put up with it a single night of your life. You deserve better than acting as a sex doll for your partner. You deserve pleasure. You deserve the chance to explore your kinks and fantasies. Sex should never be transactional.

BDSM will show you how to be freer and happier in the bedroom. These rules are a safety net for you to explore and practice sexual freedom. Don't be hung up on what society dictates is an orthodox sexual experience. Use the rules and follow your instincts. Your body knows what it wants done to it. Use your head to protect yourself.

The Keys to Being a Good Dominant Partner

To be perfectly frank, I consider myself something of an expert on D/s (Domination and submission. D/s is a truly miraculous system that has freed so many people from the responsibilities and expectations of their sexual encounters. When you enter into a sexual relationship, there's almost like this unspoken list of rules that we're all supposed to know and follow even though no one can actually conceive of the list. Traditionally the woman is just supposed to lay there as the guy ruts into her and then rolls over. It's 2019 now and women don't just have to lay there and be miserable. There's almost this secret expectation that men are supposed to take charge in the bedroom. Weirdly that set of secret societal expectations doesn't mention bringing his partner to orgasm. Problems can compound further as a couple or polyamorous relationship matures and partners fall into an unspoken routine. People want to talk about sex but are guilted and shamed by a puritanical society. Most of us want to fuck, but it's considered rude to say that during brunch. Aside from asexual people, the people who hate sex generally have never had a pleasant sexual experience and therefore hate sex for good reason. If everyone of your sexual experience's is your boyfriend or husband rutting into you like an animal without regard for your comfort, arousal, or orgasm, then sex is going to make you miserable and eventually you'll get to a point where you abstain from it altogether.

In our modern society, I think sometimes women can feel a pressure to flip the script and take charge of their sexual wellbeing. I'm all for anyone of any gender taking charge of their own sexual pleasure. It starts with exploration and courage. Though what many women find is that while they want to be treated with dignity and respect in their social and professional lives just like the rest of us, in the bedroom, they may desire something startling different.

Professional, educated, dignified women can have fantasies about being raped, degraded, and controlled and that's perfectly healthy. Sex should be exciting and breathtaking. No one is masturbating to a romp under a wool blanket with the lights off and your long underwear still on. What I hear from a lot of women in the BDSM community or those interested in it is they feel like they've cheated their way to sex and dignity. When they have theses degrading and violent fantasies, it makes them feel fake. This is where the Dominant comes in.

A Dominant is the active controlling person in the sexual relationship. For the sake of simplicity, I will refer to monogamous couple as the D/s dynamic can get very complicated for polyamorous tribes. I emphasize the sexual part of the sexual relationship. A Dominant only Dominates while in the bedroom. Female friends and acquaintances involved with BDSM frequently complain to me that they can't find a real Dom. Real Dom means a lot of different things to a lot of different people. I'm going to break down what I think it means and how it relates to safe, sane, and consensual.

For general purposes, a real Dom only Dominates during sexual activity. We'll speak later about living a D/s lifestyle, but for our purposes, we will focus strictly on the sexual component of D/s. The very first rule of D/s as a Dom is that Domination starts and ends in the bedroom. You are not your partner's boss or master. You don't get to tell them how to live their life. You are not their parent giving them ultimatums. Every real Dom knows that D/s begins and ends in the bedroom. If you can reconcile that fact, you are already ahead of 50% of the people who think they are Dom's.

Second, a Dom always carries great care and respect for their sub. This submissive is sacrificing a great amount of dignity and control to you. I don't care how rough or humiliating they want their sex to be, you will respect them as human being. They're not some whore you are taking pity on but fucking them. They have agency and value, even if they sacrifice both during sex. You are not allowed to ignore a safe-word. If you violate a safe-word by not stopping, you are a horrible human being akin to a rapist. You will never violate their hard limits. This is equally as egregious as violating the use of a safe-word. You are allowed to violate their soft limits, but must give them an opportunity to respond. You will honor any call for a red-light. I don't care how masochistic or slave-like they behave, these rules are in place to protect the mind and body of anyone participating in BDSM.

With these rules and understanding in place, you are ready to begin a D/s relationship with your partner. Start by communicating your desires for D/s with your partner. The dynamic of this kind of relationship isn't something you can wordlessly incorporate into your pre-existing relationship. Communication is key. Explain to them how this is simply a sexual dynamic and won't change your relationship with each other. This is absolutely not about taking control of the relationship but about giving you permission to take charge in this bedroom. This isn't something you can force upon your partner. If they don't want to submit to you after explaining D/s, you have to accept it. You can try other aspects of BDSM in hopes it changes their mind, but D/s only works with two willing participants.

With a willing partner, the first thing you should is make a list of limits. Both of you can absolutely have your own unique limits and both of you should respect them. D/s is not an excuse to violate your partner. Review your limits and keep them on hand if you need to. Next, create a list of things you would like to try in the bedroom. Immediate highlight any kinks that overlap with one another. Suppose your partner wants to be spanked and you want to discipline them. That is the perfect opportunity to participate in an activity you will both enjoy. Keep these lists on hand. If your partner can't think of any on the spur of the moment, it's fine to keep the list around and let them work on it. There's no pressure to instantly come up with so many things because you think you have to.

Once the lists are in place, give each other a chance to veto anything on the other list. Regardless of how compatible two people are, there will always be compromises. D/s isn't about getting the upper hand over your partner or having a bigger list where you win the competition. This is supposed to be about mutual pleasure.

Once all the preparations have been made, now it's time. There are many ways you can approach Domination. An easy place to start is with some verbal commands. Have your partner sit, kneel, lay down, take off their clothes, and/or put on lingerie. It can help to put a collar on your submissive whenever you start so they can get into a sub headspace and their body becomes ready. If they're kneeling, try ordering them to give you oral sex. Control their head with your hand or the leach attached to them. This simple act of control can be mind-blowing for some couples. D/s takes away the anxiety and expectations of your sexual encounters. If you are the Dom and your partner is the sub, you both have a strong idea of what to expect from the sexual situation. There are no more guessing or societal expectations ruining the experience. To push things further, you can have your partner present for you. Presenting means to get into a position where they can be penetrated or enveloped by you. Don't be afraid to give them a firm spanking and tell them they're a good boy or good girl if they're obeying you.

Once penetration has started, take control of the movement and give the commands. Pin them to the bed. Use verbal abuse if you feel comfortable. You are the Dominant. You are controlling the situation. Take control of them. Afterwards, you must absolutely provide your submissive with aftercare. Regardless of how intense you thought the sex was, you don't truly know the kind of emotions your partner went through. Nurture them. Hold them. Calm them with soothing words if they're upset. Aftercare is a critical part of the BDSM experience and should never ever be skipped. Even if your partner doesn't traditionally want or need aftercare, the offer must always be on the table.

Once aftercare has been fully administered to the best of your ability, now is a good time to reflect on what just happened. Discuss the things you and your partner liked and didn't like. Literally don't be afraid to take notes in your kink and fantasy journal. We live very busy lives, and if you're not having sex as regularly as you'd like to, it can be easy to forget everything that happened the last time you had sex. Be positive. This isn't a gripe situation where you get to complain about every little thing you didn't like. It's okay to ask for changes or to try something new next time, but also focus on the positives. Compliment your partner. Everyone is insecure about their sexual performance. Encouragement goes a long way to making your partner comfortable with D/s, especially if you're just starting out.

The Keys to Being a Good Submissive Partner

Regardless of gender, there is nothing wrong if you want to submit to your partner. Just because you're a man doesn't mean you have to take control of sex every time. Just because you're a woman doesn't mean you are playing into harmful gender roles or stereotypes. BDSM is about pleasure and freedom, not taking up preconceived notions of what others find sexually acceptable. It's not shameful or degrading to submit to your sexual partner. In fact, one could argue that it takes a tremendous amount of bravery to be submissive. You have to surrender control to another human being and trust that they will show you dignity and respect after sex is over. Submission is not something everyone is capable of doing. It takes a special person confident in their decisions and their sexuality.

I mentioned this in the previous section and I'll mention it here again, D/s (Domination and submission) does not carry on outside the bedroom. It can if you would like to, and I'll discuss how to do that intelligently later, but for now we are only focusing on the sexual aspects of D/s. D/s is not an excuse for your partner to start bossing you around or making decisions for you outside of the sexual encounter. If you're trying out new partners, inexperienced and uneducated Dom's can act very controlling and even degrading because they think their sexual persona is supposed to carry on in their social life even though no one ever agreed to that. Let your Dom know that the D/s is strictly sexual and ends once aftercare is over. Unless you're a masochist, and that's completely fine if you are, your Dom shouldn't make you feel bad about being submissive.

Before your BDSM session, you should discuss with your Dom your desires and expectations. Bear in mind you can't come at your Dom and say they have to do this, this, and the other thing. That's very Dominant behavior and you might not be as submissive as you are. This is called Dominating from the bottom and goes against the teachings of D/s. Remember, just because you're female, that doesn't mean you can't be Dominant. You can absolutely get penetrated by your partner and still Dominate the sexual encounter.

As a sub, what you want to do is first establish your safeword and make sure your Dom understands the stoplight system. Then you'll want to familiarize them with your limits both hard and soft. Once these rules are in place, tell your Dom the things you enjoy during sex. Maybe you like being pinned down. Maybe you like verbal abuse. You might enjoy being fondled or spanked. The more your Dom has to work with the more excited and varied your experience will be. But don't demand things from them.

Once your Dom understands the rules, your turn offs and desires, now it's time to submit. Hopefully your Dom knows a thing or two about D/s and will begin taking control of you or giving instructions. It's okay to playfully push against orders in hopes of punishment, but don't frustrate them. The entire point of submitting is you're surrendering control to your partner. If you constantly wrestle with their control, you're not respecting the role they're trying to embody. If this is your kink, make sure your partner understands you like to break rules and get punished during sex. As I've stated before, sex is not the time for surprises. Good expectations create positive experiences.

You'll slowly realize that you have tremendous amount of control as a sub during sex. Your desires and limits are vocalized and your Dom cannot do anything to violate them. In this way, you have final say in all matters. As the dominatrix Illy Hymen described, you are the dungeon master and your Dom is simply playing the game. You set the rules and parameters and your Dom always has to act within those boundaries.

During an especially intense session of D/s, you may find yourself completely overwhelmed emotionally, maybe even crying uncontrollably. This is completely normal, especially for masochists. A good D/s session can end up being one of the most intense moments of your life. Your entire life your human brain is designed to keep you in control. Except when you're asleep or intoxicated, you excerpt a massive amount of control over each moment of your life. During D/s, you let go. It's like flying down the highway on a motorcycle while someone else steers. It is an intensely freeing moment that your mind and heart might not be used to immediately. Let it out. Give in to your emotions. Cry and scream your pleasures. Let your Dom know just how much you're enjoying yourself.

After both of you are completely worn out or just need a break, aftercare is in order. After D/s, it is your Dom's responsibility to take care of your physical, mental, and emotional needs. They should tend to any physical damage from bondage or impact play. If you need to be held, it is their responsibility to hold you. If you're a masochist questioning your worth as a human being, they should tell you how much you're love and cherished until you calm down. Any Dom worth their salt will tell you that aftercare is absolutely mandatory. You have surrendered a massive amount of control and emotion to this person and now it's their job to nurture you. This is an excellent moment for you and your partner to bond. Take as much time as you need, there is no time limit on aftercare. Your Dom shouldn't rush you or say there isn't enough time. If you're going to practice D/s, then make sure you leave time for a proper amount of aftercare.

Connecting with Others

This section is specifically written for those who are single or for couples looking to introduce a new partner into their lovemaking. While dating sites are plentiful with literally millions of active users, it can be difficult to broach the subject of BDSM with a stranger. Luckily, the internet has got your back. FetLife is the first and last stop for all of you who are into the BDSM lifestyle. Think of it as an adults-only Facebook specifically for people into BDSM. There is just so much to do on FetLife that it can be truly mind boggling. There are articles and essays by people who practice BDSM. There is a messenger system to connect with other members. There is a member finder (ha, member finder, amirite?) to locate people in your area. FetLife members are constantly posting articles, pictures, and videos. There is even an events board to find festivals, lectures, and orgies in your area. While there is a $5 a month membership fee for all services, it's well worth the price if you're serious about meeting others into BDSM. If you feel you need an alternative to FetLife or just want to connect with more people, Tumblr and Reddit are also solid choices. The subreddit for the BDSM practitioner is:

https://www.reddit.com/r/bdsmcommunity. Here you can find thousands of threads discussing anything imaginable as it pertains to BDSM. Tumblr is a little harder to navigate because of the porn, but people still gather and share their ideas about the subject. Turn off your filter and try searching **d/s** on Tumblr to find thousands of blogs dedicated to BDSM.

Living the D/s Lifestyle

While I stated that D/s begins and ends inside the bedroom, there are people who choose to live it outside the bedroom, and special caveats must be made. This arrangement is possible though it requires an immense amount of patience and communication with each other. People simply aren't good at managing their relationships and surrendering control to your partner can amplify pre-existing problems. This arrangement requires two very specific people to work. In addition to both of you regularly communicating the needs of your relationship to each other, you both must have patience for mistakes. Too often couples treat their relationship as a game to be won or lost, to get one over on each other to use it as leverage against their partner the next time they make a mistake. That's psychotic and no healthy relationship can sustain such animosity forever.

D/s does take some of the problems out of modern relationships though. Each couple inevitably arrives at a point where they mutually agree on who has how much control over what in the relationship. Much of the discord in a relationship, arguably all of it, is over decision making. Who takes out the trash, who pays the cable bill, how much money to save for retirement, how to parent your child? Often both of you have an opinion that you both thinks are valid. If you're poor communicators, these small disagreements blow up into fights as a symptom of underlying resentment. If you're constantly fighting with your partner, you're probably not prepared for a D/s lifestyle. If you constantly have problems, like all relationships do, but manage them in a calm and intelligent matter, you might have what it takes.

Supposing you do have the proper relationship where effective communication solves most your problems, one of you must naturally be Dominant while the other is submissive for this lifestyle to work. It may seem counterproductive to female dignity if you're a female submissive, but that couldn't be further from the truth. True feminism is about empowering women to make their own choices, even if you don't agree with those choices. That's it. That's how complicated feminism needs to be. If you want to stay at home barefoot and pregnant and be a happy little homemaker, you're allowed to do that if it genuinely makes you happy and your relationship can afford it financially. Don't do it because you think it's expected of you by friends, family, or society, do it only if it makes you happy. On the same token, embrace your Dominant side if that's what you want. Be the breadwinner. Work the long hours then come home and run the household or let someone run you. There's no expectation on you to be a certain way. Just do what makes you happy.

There is one massive caveat though. One of you has to be submissive while the other is Dominant. In theory you can switch off on a periodic basis, but then you have long stretches of time where you're resenting their chance to be submissive or Dominant. It's one thing if you're a switch and can handle either role, but two Dominants or two submissives together won't be happy.

Now if you truly have that perfect combination of Dominant and submissive, and you're both patient communicators, you're ready to begin. The first step as always is communication. You absolutely must set down a list of goals and expectations for your D/s relationship. If you're brand new to this, I strongly urge you to establish a D/s sexual relationship over years before starting a lifestyle. With that in place, start with a handful of expectations. A simple thing could be letting the Dom decide the chores and meals. Being a Dom doesn't mean you are free from chores. Both of you should do an equal part managing your household, especially when your sub is giving up control to you. Aside from meals and chores, a simple thing you can do is decide what your sub wears every morning. Imagine how kinky it will be having your sub try on underwear or no underwear at all.

Chores, meals, and clothes are a great entry point into the D/s lifestyle. I find that for people starting out, having stop and start dates can be helpful. You may try the D/s lifestyle for a single day and see how it makes both of you feel. Try it for a week, or only do it at night. As with all elements of BDSM, start slow and move towards an intensity you are comfortable with. Don't worry about your sub finding the lifestyle degrading. Some people genuinely enjoy being degraded, while others find immense peace of mind when they're removed from the decision-making process. Being a poor decision maker is one of the common behaviors of submissive people. Subs simply aren't good at making decisions and can agonize over small decisions for several minutes if given the time. If you hate waking up every morning and having to decide what to wear, what to eat for breakfast, and what to listen to on the drive to work, this may be a great opportunity to let your partner make all those decisions for you. You may just be more submissive than you think.

PART IV

TIPS AND CHEAT SHEET

♥ ♥ ♥

And now we come to the end of the book boys and girls. I have taught you everything you need and then some to begin your BDSM journey. There's a lot to take in and you may find yourself referring back to this book for ideas and crucial information. To help you out, I have organized this chapter into tips and hot takes that you can bookmark and quickly reference when necessary.

Tips that Will Make the Start of Your BDSM Journey Easier

• Communication is key. Never hesitate to express your expectations, desires, and limits with your partner.

• Go slow. There is no hurry. Take as much time as you need to get to a place where you are comfortable but satisfied.

• Always air on the side of caution. All sex contains some inherent risk, that can be elevated when bondage and sadomasochism are brought into play. Safety is more important than adventurousness.

- Just because you're male, it doesn't mean you have to be a Dominant sadist.

- Just because you're female, it doesn't mean you have to be a submissive masochist.

- No fantasy is inherently harmful. All fantasies are safe and sane until they are acted upon.

- If you are unsure about any activity, remember the golden rule, **safe sane and consensual**.

- Use plenty of lube. Not every woman can get wet on a moment's notice. There's no shame in resorting to safe and affordable water based lubricant.

- If you're new to BDSM, start with any combination of a blindfold, spanking, and/or light verbal abuse and go from there.

- Remember the stoplight system. Green means continue, yellow means use caution, red means stop immediately.

- Respect safe-words.

- Respect limits.

Cheat Sheet

Below I have condensed the most common terms of BDSM into a glossary you can bookmark and return to as a quick reference. No list will ever truly encompass all facets of BDSM, so this cheat sheet will only cover the terms and ideas discussed in this book.

- **ABC'S**: For the purpose of safe bondage. **A**irways unobstructed, breathing easily, **C**irculation maintain, **S**cissors unhand.
- **Aftercare**: The post-coital process of tending to your partners physical, mental, and emotional needs. All sex should have aftercare available.
- •**DSM**: **B**ondage and discipline, **D**omination and submission, **S**adism and **M**asochism.
- **Bondage**: The restraint of movement or senses.
- **Bottom**: The one who is penetrated during sex.
- **Butt Plug**: A small dildo with a flared base designed to remain in your butt.
- **Caregiver**: in a DD/lg roleplay, the caregiver plays the role of the adult.
- **Cock Cage**: A male chastity belt used to prevent erections.
- **Cock Ring**: A special ring worn on your cock to create longer and harder sustained erections.
- **Consent**: Permission to do what you're about to do. The respect of limits and the safe-word.

Acknowledgment of the stoplight system. Consent can be withdrawn at any time for any reason.

- **Cuckold**: One who enjoys watching their partner have sex with others.

- **Cuffs**: Use cuffs made from leather and fabric that are cushioned. You should be able to fit two fingers comfortable between the cuff and appendage.

- **DD/lg**: A roleplay scenario where one of the participants roleplays as a child.

- **Dildo**: An artificial penis. When beginning, start small and use plenty of lube. A good dildo can be purchased for $10.

- **Discipline**: The restraint or conditioning of behavior through punishment, the threat of punishment, reward, or the promise of reward.

- **Domination**: Controlling your partner during sex within the bounds of their limits.

- **D/s**: Domination and submission.

- **Erotica**: Literotica.com contains the largest collection of free erotica on the internet.

- **Exhibitionist**: One who becomes excited or aroused when others watch them during sexual activity.

- **FetLife**: The Facebook of BDSM. The number one social media site for BDSM practitioners.

- **Fleshlight**: An artificial vagina. Expensive ones produce better results.

- **Flogger**: A small whip made of several strands of fabric used for impact play.

- **Gooning**: Abstaining from ejaculation during long sessions of masturbation. Synonymous with edging.

- **Impact Play**: Striking your partner's body to create a mixture of pain and pleasure. Combine with the stoplight system for a positive experience.
- **Little**: In a DD/lg roleplay scenario, the little roleplays as a child.
- **Masochism**: Deriving pleasure from mental, emotional, and physical pain.
- **Master**: In a D/s relationship, a master has complete control over their submissive or slave.
- **Pocket Pussy**: An artificial vagina. Expensive ones produce better results.
- **Porn**: Pornhub and Xvideos.com are safe and popular website for free porn videos. Kink.com is an excellent pay site for professionally made BDSM Porn. Sex.com hosts millions of high quality, virus free pictures.
- **Rope**: All ropes have their pro's and con's. Cotton is good for beginners. Jute rope is for experts and quite expensive.
- **Sadism**: Receiving pleasure by causing mental, emotional, and/or physical pain to others.
- **Safe, Sane, Consensual**: The golden rule of BDSM. All sex should be performed as safely as possible while not intoxicated. Consent should be exhibited at all times.
- **Slave**: A submissive who has relinquished total control to their Dom or Master.
- **Stoplight System**: A system of verbal queues used for a positive BDSM experience. Green means continue, yellow means use caution, red means stop immediately.
- **Strap-on**: A harness where the wearer can use a dildo as a cock.

- **Stroker**: An artificial vagina. Expensive ones produce better results.
- **Submission**: Giving control of the sexual situation to your partner.
- **Switch**: One who enjoys being a Dominant or submissive.
- **Top**: The one who penetrates during sex.
- **Vanilla to Kinky—The Beginner's Guide to BDSM and Kink**: The book you're reading right now, silly buns!
- **Vibrator**: A vibrating dildo. Special vibrators called prostate stimulators are designed for men.
- **Voyeur**: One who enjoys watching others.

CONCLUSION

♥ ♥ ♥

So, we've reached the end of our wonderful journey, or is it? The search for kink and knowledge is never ending. I urge you to continue this adventure into BDSM. Get all the books you can get your hands on. Talk to others in the community. Watch more porn. Yes, watch more. Move outside your comfort zone. You haven't even seen the hottest thing you'll ever see in your life. You might not have even discovered your favorite kink yet. I've been involved in BDSM for 10 years and I'm constantly discovering new and interesting things. You know they have this thing that's like a gloryhole except the girl's head goes through the hole and the guy has access to the rest of her body? It's called a reverse gloryhole and I just discovered it last year. There's so much out there. If you read erotica, try watching more porn videos. If you're on Pornhub all the time, try reading an erotic novel.

Never stop expanding your horizons. There is an entire universe of sex out there waiting to be discovered. Have you ever read taboo erotica? What about VR porn where you're in the movie? This is a brave new world of human sexuality and you're alive at the perfect time to be a part of it.

And as a closing word, if this book didn't hit you the right way, if after all this you don't find yourself intrigued, it might be possible that you're asexual and simply don't have a sex drive. You could also be dealing with serious emotional problems that prevent you from enjoying sex. Trauma, anxiety, new prescriptions, all of those things can ruin your sex drive. If you find you aren't experience interest or arousal but you want to, there are special therapists who deal solely with sexual dysfunction.

Life is too short to sit on the sideline. If you want to get in the game, you need to make the effort. Maybe BDSM just isn't for you. Maybe the vanilla stuff is all you need. And hey, that's great. As long as you are experiencing the kind of sex life that you want, that's what's important to me. I'm just glad I got to teach you something along the way. Now, get out there and enjoy yourself.

My Thanks to You

Thank you so much for reading *Vanilla to Kinky—The Beginner's Guide to BDSM and Kink*. This has been an amazing journey. Almost everything in this book, I have drawn from my own experiences, but even researching modern BDSM, I have learned so much from this book. Again, I can't believe this has finally come to fruition. Your support means the world to me. If you find yourself enjoying the book and want to help even a little, please leave a review. And I want to give a special thanks to my dominatrix friend Illy Hymen for answering my emails. She is truly the best in the business.

About the Author

Jonathan Wolf has been involved in the BDSM scene for over 12 years, but it was not until 2009 that he began studying BDSM. He identifies as an experienced Dom but also has experience switching. He is an active member in his local community and has traveled all over the country to participate in events. Jon's goal is to break the stigma and spread positivity of the BDSM lifestyle by informing others about the world of BDSM.